PARADOX OF PROFESSIONALISM:

AMERICAN NURSES IN WORLD WAR II

BY THE SAME AUTHOR

Toby Creek Chronicles

Toad and Butterfly

Works in Progress:

Miracles All 'Round Me

Codes and Band-Aids

PARADOX OF PROFESSIONALISM:

AMERICAN NURSES IN WORLD WAR II

Marsha L. Burris

Spiral Publications

Copyright © 2007 by Marsha L. Burris

Published by Spiral Publications,
Charlotte, North Carolina

Library of Congress Cataloging-in-Publication Data

Burris, Marsha L.
  Paradox of Professionalism: American Nurses in
  World War II / Marsha L. Burris
  p. cm.

  ISBN 978-0-6151-5017-8

1. Burris, Marsha L. – History of Nurses. 2. Burris,
Marsha L. – Women's History.   3. Women's
contributions to the war effort   4. Women in War   5.
Women at the Battlefront 6. Army Nursing Corps

ISBN 978-0-6151-5017-8

First U.S. Edition 2007

Copyright Acknowledgements

The author gratefully acknowledges permission
for use of the following material:

Photographs and personal diary entries
Dorothy Chinnis Light

For Dot

Her quiet courage and life of service
given for her country and
fellow human beings inspired this book.

She made a difference.

ACKNOWLEDGMENTS

The author would like to thank Donna Chinnis for technical and emotional support during the creation of this book. In addition to her encouragement every step of the process, her computer expertise has been invaluable. I would also like to thank David Beckwith who believed in me from the moment I showed him the first word of *Paradox*.

Contents

Chapter 1

Foundations of the Nursing Profession

During World War II, American women experienced new opportunities in the workplace. As the country mobilized for war, women's opportunities to participate in the war effort expanded. Along with the demands for women to fill traditional positions in low paying, low skilled, domestic and clerk jobs, more provocative nontraditional positions in civilian factories and the military opened up to women. Although nursing may be considered one of the most conventional occupations for women, its members broke through traditional barriers as they accompanied soldiers to the battlefields of Europe and Asia. American nurses worked in civilian hospitals, factories, and schools on the homefront as well as military installations overseas. Their wartime activities influenced the status and working conditions of women in the nursing profession and of women in general.

War brings the issues of nursing, and nursing education into the public arena. An examination of the nursing experience in World War II reveals one aspect of women's history. Throughout history, women have attempted to acquire equitable treatment in society and more power over decisions that affect them. They have fought for the right to gain personal fulfillment through meaningful work and a voice in decisions that concerned their work. The field of nursing provides one example of that struggle.

Like women who were mobilized for civilian jobs, nurses experienced the feeling of financial independence and pride in making a significant contribution to the war effort. Unlike the women in commercial jobs, however, nurses had numerous opportunities to influence employment policies and guidelines that affected them. One explanation for this difference may be that women in wartime jobs were newcomers to many skilled factory positions where management viewed them as a temporary aberration, useful only while the men were absent.

Meanwhile, nurses dominated their own territory and would continue to be needed by society after the war and after the men returned from war. Also, untrained women could be hired at the factories with little or no prior experience and they began producing after a fairly brief and inexpensive training period. Nurses, on the other hand, needed a formal education that required a substantial amount of investment in terms of time and personal expense in order to maintain an acceptable level of skill and knowledge. It is difficult to compare women in the civilian work force to nurses because non-nurses did not share a common identity within the female civilian workforce. Although many women in civilian jobs were active in unions pursuing fair treatment from their employers, they did not seek profession status at their respective positions as did the nurses.

Organized nursing entered the war guided by an educated and dynamic leadership elite who continued the century-old battle for professional status. To protect their investment in education and training, nursing leaders resolved to secure decision-making privileges at the workplace. They assumed that more autonomy in making decisions would produce improvements in compensation for workers. World War II could have been the catalyst that accelerated the process of professionalization for nursing, yet even after extending the limits of their skills on the battlefront, and believing they would be aptly rewarded for their contributions toward victory; nurses realized little improvement in employment conditions relative to expectations. One reason for this disappointing outcome to a sophisticated plan of occupational advancement is that, doctors, social scientists, and the general public regarded nursing as a 'semi-profession'.

Whereas the most narrow definition of a profession includes only law, medicine, the clergy and university professorship (all established in the Middle Ages and historically male dominated), semi-professions are typically dominated by females in occupations such as teaching, social work, librarianship, and nursing. Members of established professions enjoy high income, prestige, influence and autonomy as a consequence of high educational requirements.

Professions also create a self-determined and self-policing code of ethics as a result of their monopoly over their body of knowledge. Semi-professions tend to evolve from positions of assistance in male occupations. Male members then refuse to relinquish authority over the developing semi-professions because of tradition and also because of an assumption of superior judgment concerning the actions of members of the semi-professions that could reflect on the parent profession. Nursing falls into the semi-professional category because it is a predominantly female occupation and its members assist physicians in caring for patients under guidelines established and supervised by the physicians. However, since organized nursing requires formal education, demands a rigid process of licensure, and maintains a strict code of ethics, its members want to distance themselves from nonprofessionals and low status groups like secretaries, bookkeepers and sales clerks. Unable to acquire acceptance and approval from the established professions, unwilling to associate with low status occupations, and without a third acceptable alternative with which to identify, nursing occupied an ambiguous position in the world of work.

During World War II, nursing leaders recognized opportunities to use the essential nature of their skills as a bargaining tool to gain professional status. However, nurses were unable to profit from this situation because nursing leaders placed their aspirations on an unreachable goal. Rather than carving out a unique niche within the medical hierarchy from which nurses could demand advances in pay and status relative to their position in medicine, organized nursing placed their hopes of advancement on the prospects of attaining professional parity with physicians. Within the parameters of their sphere of influence, nursing leaders worked to improve educational and licensing requirements, to broaden their skill repertoire and to socialize students in a strict code of behavior, but they failed to wrest power and support from the physicians, the hospital administrators, and even many of the rank-and-file nurses themselves for professional advancement.

Although nursing encompassed a complex and diverse group of individuals, nurses entered the war years with certain shared traditions. These traditions evolved during the nineteenth century as a consequence of Florence Nightingale's considerable influence and were perpetuated by each succeeding generation of nurses as part of their code of behavior.

Florence Nightingale's influence on nursing ideology is still in evidence almost one hundred years after she made her mark on the world. The legend of Florence Nightingale is the foundation upon which nursing leaders during World War II perpetuated the gender ideology that pervaded the profession, influenced policy decisions, and set the parameters beyond which nurses could not advance.

Nursing health care, although started before the Crimean War, gained notoriety when Florence Nightingale accepted an appointment to the hospital at Scutari. While Russia and France engaged women from religious orders (called "sisters") who had been prepared to care for their armies, England used inexperienced and untrained men to care for its sick and wounded. The English Army's slow and inefficient medical system left battle casualties suffering from neglect, filth and malnutrition. Newspaper accounts of this national disgrace enraged English citizens at home; their demand for reform created the social environment conducive to change.

The crowded, filthy hospital at Scutari offended Nightingale's Victorian sensibilities. She recognized an opportunity to exercise the nineteenth century notion of gender-dictated spheres of authority in which women were endowed with qualities of gentleness, sympathy and caring. Nightingale reproduced and incorporated this middle class domestic structure within the framework of medical care-giving and the parameters for nursing were set.

Nursing became one way for middle-class women to make an acceptable transition from the private province of the home to the public sphere as few other avenues were open to middle class women who wanted to participate in public life. Although there is some debate whether Nightingale understood the theory of contagion, or Germ Theory, it is certainly true that she believed that illness and sin existed in a symbiotic relationship. She believed that cleanliness and righteous living would cure patients. Maintenance of cleanliness and attention to moral principles fell naturally within the boundaries of the nurses' craft. And one may argue that it was mere coincidence that Nightingale's penchant for cleanliness also just happened to have reduced the spread of disease which dramatically decreased the death rate.

After her return from the Crimea, Nightingale advanced her belief that a hygienic environment administered by a disciplined staff of nurses deterred disease. This belief became the foundation for developing and subsequently codifying nursing principles in her <u>Notes on Hospitals</u>. Nightingale is credited with creating a new attitude toward nursing and establishing a new acceptable occupation for women. But she based her reforms on the idea that nurses had to remain subordinate and submissive to the male physicians and hospital administrators while assuming authority only within the domain of hiring, firing, and directing the behavior of the nursing personnel. Nurses' subordination to doctors remained central as the role of the nurse evolved from private duty caretaker in individual homes, which was prevalent until World War II, to hospital employee.

War emergencies contributed greatly to the developments of medical practices associated with nursing. Since the Crimean War, when Florence

Nightingale's nursing standards became widespread, organized nursing has attempted to improve its professional status and prestige as a reward for its contributions to medicine. Past wars served as opportunities for dedicated nurses to grow and to improve their expertise by encouraging experimentation and providing a more liberal and independent environment in which to work. Nurses' actions during wartime set precedents that nursing leaders used in preparation for each succeeding war. In 1901, Congress created nurses' first official military roles. Responding to the nursing shortage during the Spanish American War, the creators hoped that the newly formed Army Nurse Corps, a branch of the Army Medical Service, would prevent future shortages of trained medical care in times of national emergencies.

Two years after the Army Nurse Corps [ANC] was created, individual states began to legislate the registration of nurses to maintain quality control. Registration established who was entitled to use the designation "registered nurse." The American Nurses Association (ANA), founded in 1911, became the largest professional women's organization in the world and fostered high standards in nursing. The ANA enacted state-wide regulations that attempted to control the practice of nursing by promoting the welfare of nurses, and protecting the public from unqualified nurses. To regulate and standardize nursing education, the association established legal approval of schools of nursing, faculty preparation and curriculum. An examining board administered examinations for certificate of licensure and granted the privilege of using the letters "R.N." to candidates who passed them successfully.

With the advent of World War I, a tremendous demand for nurses opened new fields of specialization, accelerated the educational processes already under way, and stirred the public's awareness of the importance of good nursing. For the first time in history, a carefully selected pool of nurses was available for service. In 1914, the American Red Cross sent several units of doctors and nurses to six different countries in Europe. The Red Cross, an international organization of nurses, had been founded by Jean Henri Dunant in Switzerland in 1863. Dunant was inspired by the works of Florence Nightingale and other nurses who saved lives in times of crises and worked to establish an efficient conduit of assistance and humanitarian aid to individuals in various nations enduring some emergency - natural or manmade - whose governments were unable to assist its citizens. Under conditions of war, Red Cross workers fell under the direction of the military while the organization of neutral countries gave aid to both sides of warring nations. In 1917, and again in World War II when the United States officially entered the war, the Red Cross Nursing Service became the reserve of the Army and Navy.

Nurses adopted new courses of treatment for their patients injured in World War I. Before World War I, battles were fought on a designated battlefield with a definite beginning and end. At the end of the battle, the dead and wounded were cared for; the dead were buried nearby and the wounded were brought to the hospital for medical care. In the new "trench" warfare of World War I, wounded men traveled in a continuous stream from the battlefield to the field hospital, and then to an evacuation hospital approximately 10 miles behind the lines and finally, if necessary, to a base hospital even further away from the war front. Trench warfare meant new problems and procedures with which to deal. Transporting injured soldiers from the field to the hospital took up to thirty six hours, more than ample time for soldiers' wounds to become infected or to die from exposure. In trench warfare, most wounds were caused from shrapnel, a few from bombs and almost none from bullets. Wounds to the head and face were common. For at least three years of the war, injuries from poison gases occurred. Men who survived the gas attacks often never recovered from their effects. Maintaining sanitary conditions for armies in a mobile environment proved difficult and nurses coped not only with communicable diseases and basic injuries, but also with severely damaged tissue and the unusual effects of "shell shock."

Regardless of nursing successes during the war, the prestige of the nursing profession declined after World War I ended. Demand for nursing services rose during the 1917-1918 pneumonia epidemic and again in the worldwide influenza epidemic of 1918 during a postwar shortage of trained nurses. These epidemics taxed the scarce medical and nursing resources in the civilian hospitals which meant patient care suffered in some areas. Civilians who suffered from lack of nursing care harbored negative opinions concerning the nursing profession and its achievements.

Policy-makers in organized nursing learned several lessons from past war experiences and became determined to meet the challenges of the twentieth century by becoming more educated in science and technology, and transferring that knowledge to benefit the public. The public profited the most from the development of 'prevention' as a means to combat illness. World War I served as a catalyst for the growth in this area of medical care. When 29% of World War I draftees were found physically unfit to serve in the armed forces because of preventable medical conditions, demand for public health nurses increased tremendously between 1912 and 1930 as a result.

In terms of improved education, the nursing profession began organizing schools of nursing which were independent from hospitals in the early 1920s. The first three schools of nursing, not associated with a hospital, were at Yale University, Western Reserve University, and Vanderbilt University. In the university environment, nursing curriculum emphasized the correlation between theory and clinical experience in addition to practical bedside training. In contrast, hospital training programs stressed the primary importance of bedside care over theory.

Even with advances in education, the Depression years forced eight to ten thousand graduate nurses into the ranks of the unemployed while nurses who found work often received only room and board in way of compensation. While America attempted to pull itself out of the Depression, World War II broke out in Europe. Over a year and a half before the United States formally entered the war, American nursing leaders began making preparations. Nurses who planned and crafted policy within the organizational hierarchy built upon the advances attained during the previous war. Many of these nurses in leadership positions had participated in

World War I in an official capacity. They brought with them both a strong military tradition and a philosophy based on Nightingale's Victorian traditions of separate spheres for doctors and nurses, self-sacrifice and severe self-discipline. Indeed most of the women leading the profession had been raised in traditional Victorian families that advocated a strong sense of service in the community.

The most influential of these nurses in leadership positions who determined the direction of nursing during World War II were Julia C. Stimson, Julia O. Flikke, Florence A. Blanchfield, Katherine J. Densford, Stella Goostray, Mary Beard, Alma Haupt, Annie Goodrich, and Mary Roberts.

Julia C. Stimson, President of the American Nursing Association from 1938 to 1944 had been a career officer in the Army Nurse Corps and served in France during World War I. Like so many of the other leaders, Stimson returned to active duty after retirement and brought with her a lifetime of knowledge and expertise to the war effort. Stimson was born in 1881 and came from a family that placed great importance on higher education, service to others, and the right of all family members to pursue a career. Stimson graduated from Vassar College in 1901. After graduation, she attended the New York Hospital Training School at Cornell, at the encouragement of Annie Goodrich, the nursing school's superintendent. Upon completion of her nursing degree, Stimson accepted the superintendent's position at the nursing school at Washington University Hospital in St. Louis. At Washington University she completed graduate degrees in sociology, biology, and education.

In 1917, when the United States entered the war, Stimson enlisted and volunteered for duty in France where she served as the director of a Red Cross-sponsored hospital. Stimson remained in France until six months after the end of the war. After returning home, Stimson became the Superintendent of the Army Nurse Corps where she focused on improving the status of nurses through re-organization and enlightened personnel practices until her retirement in 1937. In 1942, the Army recalled Stimson from retirement to active duty to assist in recruiting nurses for World War II. During the war, she served as president of the American Nurses Association and was instrumental in setting policy for recruiting and directing nurses to meet the challenges of war.

Julia O. Flikke followed Stimson as the sixth Superintendent of the Army Nurse Corps from 1937 until 1943, first with the rank of Major and subsequently rising to the rank of Colonel. After Flikke became widowed in 1912 at the age of 33, she attended Augustana Hospital Training School in Chicago. Upon graduation in 1915, she pursued postgraduate work in administration and nursing education at the Teachers College, Columbia University. In 1918, after teaching for two years, Flikke enlisted in the Army Nurse Corps to serve in France. Between the wars, Flikke served at military installations in the United States, the Philippines and in China. At Walter Reed Hospital in Washington, D.C., Flikke served as the principal chief nurse from 1922 to 1934. From 1927 through 1937, she also served as Assistant Superintendent of the Army Nurse Corps. In 1937, Flikke accepted the appointment to Superintendent. Two years later, when war broke out in Europe, Flikke began the process of expanding the 625-member Army Nurse Corps. She actively campaigned for commissioned status for nurses in the Army, establishing a proper place for the corps as a permanent part of the Army.

During her career, Flikke attained only the relative rank of Colonel. Relative rank meant nurses did not enjoy the same privileges of authority as other military women and men of the same rank and grade. Flikke's efforts bore fruit when her successor became the first woman to receive a regular commissioned rank of Colonel. Before leaving office, Julia Flikke established a standardized training program to prepare nurses for overseas duty and wrote Nurses in Action in 1943 to educate the public about the responsibilities of the army nurse.

Flikke's successor was Florence A. Blanchfield, a 61-year-old career Army nurse who continued the campaign to improve nurses' status in the Army from 1943 until her retirement in 1947. Blanchfield had studied nursing at Southside Hospital Training School for Nurses in Pittsburg, Pennsylvania and pursued diverse educational interests throughout her active career. After gaining experience in executive administration in civilian hospitals prior to World War I, Blanchfield joined the ANC in 1917 and sailed to war-torn France where she served as chief nurse at a camp hospital. A brief return to civilian nursing at the end of World War I proved unfulfilling and Blanchfield reentered the ANC to serve successively at various Army hospitals and military bases in the United States, the Philippines, and China. At the time the United States entered World War II, Blanchfield held a key position at Walter Reed Hospital in Washington, D.C. from which she moved into the position vacated by Flikke. Blanchfield brought educational and practical experience to the highest position in the ANC during the war years.

Katherine J. Densford succeeded Stimson as president of the ANA in 1944 and served in that capacity for four years. Densford also grew up in a family that emphasized the importance of education, service and occupational opportunities for women. Although Densford earned both B.A. and M.A. degrees in history and enjoyed a career in teaching, World War I influenced her to pursue nursing education. Densford attended the Vassar Training Camp and ultimately graduated from the nursing program at the University of Cincinnati. Densford worked in the field of public health until 1930 when

she accepted the directorship of the University of
Minnesota School of Nursing from which she retired
in 1959. From 1934 until 1948, Densford also served
on the ANA board of directors; twice during World
War II as its president. After the war ended,
Densford continued to work toward establishing
collective bargaining for nurses, improving the
economic welfare of the members of the nursing
profession, and integrating minority groups into all
levels of the nursing organization.

Stella Goostray, President of the National
League of Nursing Education (NLNE) worked to
establish the Nursing Council for National Defense
and served on its board of directors from 1940-1942
when the council reorganized to become the National
Nursing Council for War Service. Goostray then
served as its president until 1946 bringing with her a
strong dedication to the professionalization of
nursing through particularly high standards in nurse
education. Goostray earned a B.S. degree from
Teachers College of Columbia University in 1926
and an M.Ed. degree from Boston University in 1933,
both after completing the nursing program at the
Children's Hospital School of Nursing in Boston in

1919. Through her participation on various committees in World War II, Goostray worked to maintain gains made by nurses through higher standards of education. Throughout her career, Goostray remained determined to elevate the status of nurses in the military.

Mary Beard, Director of the American Red Cross Nursing Service (ARCNS), chaired the subcommittee on nursing for the Federal Council of National Defense which was responsible for the education, procurement, and distribution of military and civilian nurses. Beard graduated from the New York Hospital of Nursing in 1903 and contributed significantly to the field of public health nursing, especially through the National Organization of Public Health Nursing (NOPHN) which she was instrumental in founding. Because of her extensive studies of nursing practices in Europe, China, Japan, and other countries, Beard's participation in the American Red Cross Nursing Service and the Council of National Defense was extremely valuable.

Alma Haupt played a similar role to Beard's while serving as nursing consultant and executive secretary of the nursing subcommittee of the Office of Defense Health and Welfare Services in Washington, D.C. Haupt, like Beard, made many contributions to public health nursing. Following a family tradition of community and religious leadership, Haupt used her degrees in physical education and nursing education from the University of Minnesota to improve the health and social welfare of the urban poor in Minneapolis. In 1924, Haupt was invited to help develop American ideas of public health service organizations in war-torn Austria. Her knowledge of the effects of war on civilians was exceptionally useful in Haupt's role in the Office of Defense, Health and Welfare during World War II where she coordinated the activities of nurses from twelve governmental agencies.

Annie Goodrich served on planning committees and established the Army School of Nursing during World War I. During World War II, Goodrich became a consultant to the U.S. Public Health Service and in that capacity, helped develop the Cadet Nurse Corps, a government sponsored school of nursing. Goodrich stressed that nursing, and the medical profession, were equally important to each other - independent and interdependent. As a young woman, Goodrich attended private schools in the United States and abroad until her father's illness decreased the family fortunes. Motivated by the need to support herself, Goodrich chose nursing in 1890 as one of the few desirable careers open to women. Goodrich completed her education at New York Hospital's Training School for Nurses and entered hospital administration as superintendent of nurses at New York Postgraduate Hospital. In this position, she worked for many improvements in nursing, including raising entry requirements into nursing schools, expanding the curriculum and increasing clinical experience, creating compulsory state registration of nurses, establishing licensing examinations and producing graduates with a sense of high professional standards. With this focus, Goodrich developed the concept for the Army School of Nursing during World War I to maintain standards while producing more nurses for the war effort.

In the inter-war years, Goodrich participated in the Rockefeller Foundation study of nursing education in 1918 and the Goldmark Report in 1923. At the request of the Rockefeller Foundation in 1935, she toured European countries to observe their hospital systems. During World War II, Goodrich once again used her background and experience to establish the Cadet Nurse Corps as a response to the enormous need of nurses to serve in the Army.

And finally, Mary Roberts served her profession for 28 years (1921 - 1949) as editor of *The American Journal of Nursing*. Roberts' particular interest was in nursing journalism and her message remained constant - only a well-educated nurse can offer expert care to the patient. Coming from a working class background in a company town in Michigan, Roberts attended the Jewish Hospital Training School for Nurses in Cincinnati, Ohio against her father's wishes. She excelled in school and graduated in 1899 at the age of 22. During World War I, Roberts recruited nurses for the American Red Cross to serve in the Army reserve and volunteered for active duty herself in July 1918. Roberts served as chief nurse and director of the Army School of Nursing at Camp Sherman, Ohio.

After the war, at age 42, Roberts entered the Teachers College, Columbia University to earn a B.S. degree and a diploma in nursing school education. Upon completion of this part of her education,

Roberts accepted the appointment of editor of *The American Journal of Nursing*. As editor, Roberts concentrated on bringing the needs of individual nurses together with the demands of the profession and provided a forum of dialogue between the two concerns.

Roberts' knowledge and concern for the various aspects of nursing became useful during World War II in the capacity as a consultant for the recruiting agencies and various committees of the American Nurses Association. Additionally, Roberts wrote the classic history of nursing in 1954 titled American Nursing: History and Interpretation.

Members of this leadership elite had much in common with each other. Most of them were born during the late nineteenth century and were raised with a strong sense of service, duty, and social obligation learned both at home and as part of their formal education. To be successful in public life, they chose careers over marriage. And each woman had participated in World War I which directed her way of thinking and consequently the course of nursing during World War II.

To address nursing preparedness in the U.S., the American Nurses' Association, the National League of Nursing Education, and the National Organization for Public Health Nursing, represented by Stimson, Goostray, Beard, and Roberts, held their first joint convention in May 1940. Their main objectives were to preserve control over nursing by determining how nurses would be used in the war and to orchestrate all nursing activities related to the war. To achieve these goals, the nursing leadership established the Nursing Council of National Defense which became the National Nursing Council for War Service in 1942. The National Nursing Council represented the ANA, the National League of Nursing Education, the National Organization for Public Health Nursing, the Red Cross Nursing Service, the Federal nursing services, the Association of Collegiate Schools of Nursing, and the National Association of Colored Graduate Nurses.

While dynamic personalities within the nursing leadership influenced the profession's directions, developments and improvements in medicine and technology worked as an outside, objective and impersonal force guiding nursing to new levels of proficiency and skill. Manufacturers constructed operating room furniture, cabinets, lab equipment, kitchen and laundry fixtures, basins, jars, utensils and trays from lighter, stronger and more sanitary stainless steel. Improved casters meant more mobility and easier handling of patients, and more efficient distribution of food, equipment and supplies. Technical improvements reduced response times for retrieving therapeutic apparatus and other supplies, and relieved some of the physical strain on the nurses, allowing them to concentrate on their medical duties. Brighter and cooler illumination in the operating room, emergency auxiliary power generators, signaling devices for patient communication with the nurses' station, and air conditioners created a more comfortable working environment in the hospitals. Over-bed tables for holding patients' food trays, adjustable beds and backrests, removable side rails, and cubicle screening curtains in multi-patient rooms provided patients with comfort, safety and privacy and made the time nurses spent in attendance with each patient more efficient.

Technological advances and an increased repertoire of effective drugs developed prior to the war improved survival rates of the wounded and ill men during World War II. The first sulfa miracle drug, Sulfanilamide, became available in 1936 in time to treat bacterial infections sustained during the war. In 1939, a London physician, Dr. Alexander Fleming, provided the medical profession with the miracle antibiotic, penicillin. DDT effectively eliminated insects and rodents, the carriers of malaria and typhus. Pharmaceutical companies made great strides in tropical medicine, too, by using Atabrine as a substitute for quinine. Also, antihistamines, cortisone and ACTH relieved allergic and other respiratory conditions. Through new and improved techniques, blood replacement became standardized and blood banks developed efficient methods for handling the processing, storage, and distribution of whole blood and blood plasma.

Even with considerable advances in education and technology, and the opportunity to display its nursing skills during World War II, the nursing profession remained unable to achieve the elevated status toward which it worked. The vital importance of their services in the war effort convinced nurses that their contributions were essential to national security in particular and to the basic health and welfare of American society in general. During their actual participation in war, nurses found themselves well-prepared for their duties because of their comprehensive and strict nursing training program, a program steeped in the traditions of Florence Nightingale's reforms. Within the parameters where nurses maintained control - that is, in education and registration and certification - they improved nursing standards significantly and made advances that even tested the boundaries. But outside their sphere of control - in hospital administration and personnel policy-setting positions - nursing leaders were unable to make substantial gains, and military nurses who returned from years at the front believed that they deserved more equitable treatment in the workplace.

Nurses wanted opportunities to use their skills fully and to have access to higher wages and better benefits. But nursing leaders subscribed to the Victorian notion that the nursing profession was a calling. They held that nursing care should be under the direction of physicians and that salary, although important, should not be the determining factor for choosing nursing as one's vocation. Their devotion and allegiance to this nineteenth century ideology created many of the limits to professionalization beyond which they could not break. Within that context, policies asking for better personnel practices in the workplace lacked the force of aggressive demands especially in terms of wage compensation.

The characteristics that guaranteed their successes in the war were the very qualities that prevented nurses from qualifying for full-fledged professional status. This paradox developed during World War II as nursing leaders struggled to appease the male power structure in the federal government, in the armed forces, in medicine and in the hospitals. This process created conflicts and incompatibilities in nurses' attempts to professionalize the nursing field while the male power structure exploited nurses' skills for the war effort. How nursing leaders dealt with these tensions produced by the interaction of a female-dominant occupation with the traditional male preserves is the theme of the remainder of this book. In the following chapters, I investigate the actions initiated by organized nursing during the war and how those actions affected the profession as it entered the postwar era. Nursing leaders were aware that every effort should be made to thwart another postwar decline in public confidence and support but they were met by many obstacles that confronted them in their wartime efforts to improve their profession. Women like Stimson, Flikke, Blanchfield, Densford, Goostray, Beard, Haupt, Goodrich, and Roberts enthusiastically embraced the challenge of wartime nursing as an opportunity to advance their professional standing in the medical field in terms of wages, image, status, education, and duties.

In structuring this study, I chose to focus on nurses who experienced war through the Army Nurse Corps rather than the Navy Nurse Corps because the Army nurses were a greater presence overseas than Navy nurses who were typically stationed stateside. Army nurses who served overseas had the opportunity to exceed the limits often associated with traditional female roles and nurses' roles. My sources include published memoirs, autobiographies, and popular magazine articles. I also use editorials, articles and letters to the editor in *The American Journal of Nursing*. A final resource of importance is a personal interview with Dorothy Chinnis Light substantiated by excerpts from the diary she kept daily while overseas. My written correspondence with Chinnis' chief nurse in the Army Nurse Corps during the war reflects one leader's personal point of view. Admittedly, each of these sources has an agenda that reflects the background and history of the individual or organization. Documents created by participants tend to be flattering to their creators. Nevertheless, examination of these materials provides the investigator with a glimpse into the administration of policy by the nursing elite and the consequences of those policies on the individual rank-and-file nurses.

Chapter Two

When Uncle Sam Calls: Meeting the Needs of the Army Nurse Corps

The United States government considered nursing a strategic defense skill during World War II and declared nursing an essential part of military service. As in previous wars, nursing leaders seized this opportunity to pursue a higher professional standing in the medical field. They believed that failure to meet the challenges of war would damage their chances to professionalize. Since the late nineteenth century, an "articulate and self-conscious elite" worked to make nursing a respectable occupation for middle class and working class women. Even though organized nursing tried to professionalize its field by seeking public legitimacy through licensure, employment standards and educational credentials, the field of nursing contained problematic characteristics that prevented it from becoming a full-fledged profession comparable to medicine. Professions enjoy autonomy, self-accountability, privileges of confidences and secrecy, and the right of members to determine their own professional standards and set their own fees. Members in a profession also establish minimum qualifications for its practice, enforce rules and codes of behavior and continually seek to raise the status of the profession in general society. Nursing possesses many of these qualities and therefore its members want to be considered within the province of the professions. However, nurses are powerless to act independently of physicians causing difficulties for the nursing elite who sought to elevate their status.

Another problem inherent in nursing with which the nursing elite had to contend was its feminine nature. In fact, one historian wrote that "women's dominance in nursing nearly equals our monopoly on motherhood." The burdens of a traditionally female occupation striving for professional status were many. Like other women's occupations, nursing had to overcome low wages, an obligatory deference to male superiors, which in this case included physicians and hospital administrators, and an association with menial or dirty work. Unlike other occupations in which women participated, however, nursing leaders were able to play active roles in shaping their work place while representing an "elite" among working women. That is, nursing was considered by society as one of the more desirable jobs for women, one in which women who desired a higher education for themselves and who had been influenced by a strong service tradition could dedicate their efforts.

Nineteenth century nursing schools actively pursued upper-class women as students. Nursing school administrators thought character was more important than skills, and upper or middle class women were believed to have more potential for acceptable character than the lower or working class women. Since many duties performed by nurses resemble those of low-status domestic drudgery, administrators found it difficult to attract "desirable women" into positions other than for administrative positions and positions in education. Essentially, nursing schools fostered two educational tracks: applied and administrative. By directing the student nurses into one direction or the other, administrators created a two-tiered hierarchy.

While at school, students received instruction in cultural values equal to or surpassing that given for nursing skills. Many of the women interested in nursing felt a strong attraction to idealism and felt that nursing for them was a calling. Both of these qualities were important components in comprising the boundaries of a semi-profession. Nursing, in short, was and is a very attractive and 'legitimate' career choice for women.

Organized nursing confronted the first and immediate challenge of World War II by working to fill the quota of nurses requested by the military. The military needed nurses to complement the fighting forces deploying overseas and to staff medical facilities at training posts and military hospitals at home. Instead of facilitating the process of obtaining recruits, Army policy placed major restrictions on recruitment efforts. The Army required the Nursing Corps to be totally voluntary, and it demanded the pool of eligible recruits to be limited to young, white, single females. Also, the Army expected eligible recruits to be won away from competing industries or other positions within the military.

One problem associated with an all-volunteer nurse corps concerned lack of news about the activities of nurses already in the military. Security restrictions put a premium on secrecy and hampered the flow of information released about the circumstances under which service nurses who were already stationed in combat areas worked. This dilemma seriously handicapped recruiters early in the war since lack of information created an air of mystery and consequently a fear of volunteering for service.

Lack of information also encouraged rumors, forcing recruiters to address the issue of safety for nurses in active duty. Many nurses entertained the notion of volunteering for service but shared the concern and reservations of their families about personal safety. In response, nursing leaders promised that *Uncle Sam* rewards those who enter the Army Nurse Corps by constant and vigilant planning for their futures and for the maximum safety attainable in wartime." Despite assurances of their safety, however, many nurses suffered casualties of war similar to those suffered by the men. Ironically, after publicity began to flow about the activities and movements of the Army Nurse Corps, recruitment rates increased.

Another problem with recruitment was that the armed forces wanted only young, white, middle class women as part of the nursing corps. Initially, to be eligible for a commission in the Army Nurse Corps, the Army required candidates to be female, forty years old or younger, single, physically fit, a graduate of an accredited school of nursing, and a member of the American Nurses Association. Although black nurses met the qualifications for Corps eligibility, they were not actively recruited for Foreign Service and consequently served state-side at predominantly black installations. Although black nursing leaders worked throughout the war to challenge the racist policies created in the United States Army and Navy, concessions came slowly at a time when demand for nurses appeared critical. A policy declaring an end to quotas and exclusions emerged finally in January, 1945.

Similar to Florence Nightingale's Victorian ideals concerning the 'right type' of women for nursing, the military also wanted nurses who would not question the sexual division of labor in military operations and would share an inclination toward self-sacrifice. Although non-white nurses shared ideals comparable to white nurses, the military suffered from the same structural racism found in society. Furthermore, since most of the soldiers who would require care were white - and in order that nurses could fulfill their morale-building and nurturing role to these men - the corps wanted recruits who resembled soldiers' wives, sweethearts and mothers - in other words: young and white.

Overcoming these restrictions required a concerted effort among the nursing elite that primarily included: Julia Stimson, President of the American Nurses Association (ANA); Stella Goostray, President of the National League of Nursing Education (NLNE); Mary Beard, Director of the American Red Cross Nursing Service (ARCNS);

and Mary Roberts, Editor of *The American Journal of Nursing* (AJN).

———

Organized nursing competed with civilian industrial jobs and other military positions for women workers. Nursing especially wanted to attract women with college degrees in science. Many of those women accepted teaching jobs, jobs as laboratory technicians, or jobs as industrial chemists - all of which offered more attractive wages than she could earn in traditional women's occupations. Technical institutes like Rensselaer Polytechnic Institute in New York allowed women to enroll in their programs for the first time during World War II. Female engineers found opportunities working for companies like Curtiss-Wright, Monsanto, DuPont, and Standard Oil. Even Wall Street investment firms employed women as analysts and statisticians.

Propaganda used to mobilize women in the civilian work force paralleled military recruitment efforts. Although industry sought women to fill nontraditional jobs, advertisement for those jobs used domestic comparisons. For example, one campaign stated that working in a war-related industry was, "pleasant and as easy as running a sewing machine, or using a vacuum cleaner." Propagandists designed their message to exalt factory work as attractive and alluring, thereby avoiding having to question conventional assumptions about women's roles.

In an attempt to win workers away from competing employment opportunities, nursing recruiters stressed the traditional nature of their profession. In recruitment propaganda, recruiters emphasized the intrinsic rewards of nursing over economic remuneration of other work and stressed the postwar job security only women in a woman's occupation would enjoy. Recruiters played upon the general assumption that all women ultimately wanted to become wives and mothers, and that a career in nursing offered incomparable preparation for homemaking in contrast to industries such as the laboratories, factories, radio stations, and flying fields that did not teach domestic skills. From the very start, recruiters placed more emphasis on how the nurturing aspects of nursing would help the Army rather than stressing the professional medical skills nurses would acquire under wartime conditions.

One of the most difficult problems nursing leaders encountered was something over which they had no control; inconsistent and erroneous quotas. In spite of the problems created by using all volunteers, adhering to restrictions on class, sex and race, and competing with other jobs, nursing leaders on the planning committee accepted the recruitment numbers from the Surgeon General's office without question even when the numbers were grossly over-inflated and unsubstantiated. The American Red Cross Nursing Service assumed the official responsibility for surmounting the difficulties and supplying a pool of qualified nurses to the Army for their Nurse Corps.

Although the American Red Cross functioned as a recruitment agency for the Army Nurse Corps, individual nurses could apply directly to the Army Nurse Corps for commissions. However, nurses typically joined the First Reserves of the Red Cross and agreed to serve in the Army or Navy only during the crisis of war.

To maintain a constant flow of nurses for military service, the Red Cross recruited on three different but interrelated levels. On one level, nursing leaders directed their campaign toward attracting female high school students into nurse education programs. On another level, educators sought to interest current nursing students in volunteering for military service upon graduation. And on a third level, recruiters solicited registered nurses who were skilled and available for military service immediately.

Nurses found themselves in demand in many areas. The military needed nurses in training camps at home and at the battlefields abroad. Civilian hospitals needed to maintain a nursing staff sufficient to serve public health needs. And finally, nursing schools needed educators to teach additional programs for the young women who recruiters hoped would become nursing students. The military would only accept graduate or registered nurses with a 1-A classification. The Armed Services gave a 1-A rating

to nurses who fulfilled all the requirements of
military service, and therefore a nurse with a 1-A
rating was the first-choice candidate for recruiting
purposes.

To fill the positions vacated by nurses
enlisting in the military, civilian hospitals called upon
older nurses, nurses with dependents, married nurses
and auxiliary personnel. Public relations campaigns,
created by the American Red Cross, targeted young
women in high school, college and private industry.
Messages in advertising campaigns exploited the
glory of the nursing profession. Advertisers also
placed responsibility for the fighting man's welfare
on nurses' shoulders should proper medical care be
unavailable to them.

As a result of their enlightened foresight, nursing
leaders began expanding their programs before the
U.S. formally entered the war. They planned for an
increase in enrollment of 50,000 students for the
1941 academic year and 55,000 more students in
1942. Meeting this quota was difficult because it

required increased funding for education. Federal assistance in the form of nursing education subsidies amounted to $1,250,000 in 1941 but reached over $176,000,000 during the course of the war which made educational and training programs more accessible to students with modest means.

Federal assistance funds helped to increase student enrollment in programs such as basic instruction in undergraduate schools of nursing, postgraduate instruction in specialized fields of nursing, and refresher courses for retired or inactive nurses. The federal government's investment of such a large amount of money in nursing education demonstrated the importance of nursing to the nation's destiny. In addition to federal monies, women's clubs and other groups offered scholarships to individual nursing students to further defray the costs of education for individual students. Some women's clubs that provided scholarships to young women entering the nursing field included Women of the Moose, Rotary Clubs, Auxiliary of the AMA, and America Legion Auxiliary.

As public relations programs attracted more students into the nursing field, expanding the teacher population became necessary. The National Nursing Council strongly urged educators to retain their teaching positions rather than volunteer for war service. During World War I educators had been encouraged to abandon their posts and move into nursing the troops, a mistake that nursing leaders in World War II intended to avoid.

Expanding education programs gained momentum in early 1942 after Pearl Harbor. The National Nursing Council for War Service, the coordinating agency through which all other nursing organizations acted as a unit, organized and implemented a nationwide mobilization campaign directed toward the individual woman and her community. The Council targeted two populations of young women it hoped to attract:

1. College hopefuls
2. Current students of nursing

Recruiting young women into educational programs meant increasing contacts with high schools. Using young nurses to speak and appeal to other young women became a successful strategy in soliciting nursing school enrollees. Nursing leaders urged graduate nurses to recruit at least one new student each through personal contact. The National Nursing Council created professional recruiting kits containing a list of suggestions for addressing high school and college students, a book and film list from the Nursing Information Bureau, reprints of recruitment broadcasts by notable persons with social standings, and recent reprints from *Mademoiselle*, *Harper's*, and *School and College Placement*. These materials, along with posters and displays in department stores, were also used for general promotional purposes.

To educate members of the community about nursing school opportunities, local organizers set up exhibits and displays at county fairs and other local gatherings. State nursing council speakers spoke before women's clubs and auxiliaries as members of the local Red Cross organizations worked to fill the quotas. While holding demanding full-time nursing positions, these volunteer recruiters worked far into the evenings assisted by volunteers from parent-teacher associations and other organizations contacting potential recruits.

Volunteers from nursing schools attended committee meetings and speaking engagements and tirelessly visited various communities trying to persuade young women to become interested in the nursing profession. Other avenues for reaching potential nursing students included distributing leaflets, publishing articles in sorority and academic magazines, and broadcasting radio spot announcements. Radio and magazine campaigns, created and implemented by the War Advertising Council of the Office of War Information, yielded a wealth of responses requesting information about enrollment in nursing classes. NBC network radio programs, sponsored by the American Red Cross, included shows titled "That They Might Live" and "March of Mercy" in which Helen Hayes, Margaret Sullivan and other well-known stars dramatized the urgency of the nursing service.

To recruit students enrolled in nursing programs for the Reserves, nursing leaders used one-to-one contact and word-of-mouth. The Recruitment Committee of the Nursing Council prepared pamphlets, posters and bulletins and sent them to selected nursing schools for use in recruitment.

Students were a captive audience and teachers appealed to their sense of duty and moral obligation inside the classroom and out. Likewise, the Recruitment Committee called for nurse graduates with leadership qualities and for young followers with courage of mythical proportions to join the war effort. Messages published in professional journals stressed each nurse's duty and responsibility to join the military rather than appealing to the skilled professionalism of the trained nurse.

Recruiters used massive appeals to patriotism *and* to guilt incorporated in passages like:

- *As the Army nurse, your work is more than noble, it is glorious.*

- *If we fail to assist them, men will die in the service of our country who need not have died.*

- *Recruitment lags. Can it be that the apathy of nurses themselves is in some way responsible?*

- *The individual alibis we shall have to live with hereafter will be extremely uncomfortable if we make narrow or selfish decisions now.*

- *Each and every nurse must accept the challenge of '43. Otherwise the Allied Nations will win the war, but we shall have lost the soul of the profession.*

After being moved to action, either through guilt, a sense of duty and adventure, or financial expectations, a nurse's next step would be to apply to the secretary of the nearest local committee of the Red Cross Nursing Service for a commission in the Army or Navy.

In addition to patriotism and a sense of duty, many women did enter the Army Nurse Corps for economic reasons and in response to the effects that the Depression had on job availability. For example, Edith Aynes entered military life as a reserve nurse in 1934. Aynes came from a mid-western working class background. She chose a nursing career against her mother's wishes who considered the nursing profession unsuitable for her daughter because "nursing is emptying bedpans and doing other disgusting things for people." After much searching, Aynes could not find employment. Even the hospital where she trained would not hire its graduates. Most hospitals preferred to employ only student workers because of the savings in salary expense. Private duty nursing typically absorbed the new graduates but only a few private duty positions were available during the Depression. The military, therefore, provided an outlet in which Aynes and other nurses could use their skills and earn a living.

Some nurses volunteered only out of a sense of duty, though. For example, Theresa Archard (from Massachusetts) answered the call for nurses from a local Red Cross chapter in January 1941 as expansion efforts began to accelerate. She initially enlisted for one year of active duty but after the bombing of Pearl Harbor, she and her friend, Dorothy Pridham, volunteered for foreign duty and reenlisted for the duration of the war. "Duration-plus-six-months" was the standard contractual agreement between First Reserve nurses in the Army Nurse Corps and the Army during the war. Archard and Pridham asserted their independence by going overseas voluntarily. In an environment where women typically found it difficult to justify so much freedom, they were afraid to tell their parents that they made the decisions on their own. Instead they both agreed that each would tell her parents, "We're

G.I. now... the government can do as it pleases with us."

In April 1942, at age twenty-two, Dorothy Chinnis from Ravenel, South Carolina enlisted in the First Reserves. Chinnis responded to a gentle but firm suggestion from her former nursing school supervisor who told her, "if you want to help out your fellow man... the war is the best place to do it." Originally, Chinnis applied to the Navy Nurse Corps only to be rejected for being underweight and having slightly imperfect vision. The Navy forwarded her application to the Army as part of its policy. The Army then invited Chinnis to serve with the Army Nurse Corps. She accepted and applied for foreign duty. After being stationed at Fort Jackson, S.C. for one year to the day, Chinnis joined her unit that deployed to North Africa in April 1943. She, like Archard and Pridham, never told her mother that the decision to go overseas was entirely voluntary.

Chinnis' Chief Nurse in North Africa, Dorothy Parsons, had joined the Army Nurse Corps in December 1940 during the early days of expansion. The Corps mailed Parsons a letter and invited her, as a member of the Red Cross, to join.

The Red Cross had not previously called on Parsons to serve in any other emergency so she felt duty-bound to accept the invitation. She received a promotion to Assistant Chief Nurse in 1942 at Camp Shelby, Mississippi where she worked in the Administration office. Parsons left for overseas duty in 1943 with Chinnis and the rest of the unit which was typical of the acceleration of U.S. troop participation in the war.

Another force that prompted nurses to action was the crisis at Pearl Harbor. Pearl Harbor provided nursing leaders with the drama necessary to motivate uncommitted young nurses to volunteer for military service out of a sense of adventure coupled with patriotism. *The American Journal of Nursing*, the official voice of the American Nursing Association, directed a considerable amount of space to the war. *The Journal* published articles and editorials written by nursing leaders at home, and personal accounts written by nurses at the battlefront. Typically, these articles adopted a solicitous tone pleading for volunteers to offer their specialized skills to the service of their country. *The Journal* often used personal appeals and words of inspiration issued by women of influence. This was a useful and successful recruiting tool. Even Mrs. Eleanor Roosevelt made the following plea from her summer flower garden in Washington:

> *I ask for my boys what every mother has a right to ask - that they be given full and adequate nursing care should the time come when they need it. Only you nurses who have not yet volunteered can give it... You must not forget that **you have it in your power to bring back some who otherwise surely will not return.***

> *(Emphasis Mrs. Roosevelt's)*

Whereas the American Red Cross actively recruited nurses for the military, the Nursing Council determined that as a voluntary agency, the Red Cross should not have the additional responsibilities of placing nurses into eligibility classifications. The Council, therefore, delegated this task to the Nursing Division of the Procurement and Assignment Service (P&AS) under the War Manpower Commission. The

P&AS was endowed with the advantages of federal prestige and federal financing that the American Red Cross did not have.

The P&AS held their first production conference in September 1943 when it began assigning quotas for recruitment for military service based on the stated needs of the Army and Navy. The P&AS functioned under two guidelines:

1. To procure nurses to meet the needs of the armed forces, having due consideration for civilian nursing needs.

2. To bring about equitable distribution of nurses in order to maintain the best possible nursing service for the civilian population and non-military governmental services.

Although women were not subject to the Selective Service Act, the Nursing Division of the P&AS acted rather aggressively and ingeniously in its recruitment of female nurses. They located professional nurses and classified them in accordance with their indispensability in civilian positions or in accordance with their availability for military service if they held nonessential positions. Through these efforts, they discovered evidence of unfair personnel practices toward nurses in civilian hospitals in terms of varying lengths of shifts, pay and workplace expectations but these problems would not be addressed until the nurses who served in the armed services returned home and demanded better working conditions.

Recruiters scoured every conceivable area for qualified nurses whom they could persuade to answer Uncle Sam's call. Appealing to hospital administrators to release staff nurses who were eligible to fill positions in the armed forces, nursing leaders implied that selfishness and laziness on the part of the administrators compelled them to retain the nurses they now employed.

To fill vacancies created by nurses who volunteered for military service, recruiters sent out a call to married and older nurses to contribute their services to civilian hospitals in some capacity. In the civilian work force, employment policies that discriminated on the basis of marital status originated during the Depression. Advocates of these procedures blamed married women for taking jobs away from men. Policies in nursing that barred married women from employment were based on competing loyalties. Hospital administrators and

62

school superintendents viewed marriage as an objectionable trait for nurses. Nurses endured such strict discipline, including but not limited to living arrangements, that if they were married, the administrators were afraid they would be in competition with the husband in directing the nurses' lives and capturing their loyalty. When a woman's obligation to husband and family competed with the work place for her energies, home life usually won. When the pool of available single women vanished, these same policies became important issues for reconsideration.

This divided loyalty was also part of the problem why nursing was destined to remain a semi-profession. Many nurses who were ineligible for a position because of the age and marriage restrictions criticized the artificially created restrictions arguing, "A nurse is a nurse regardless of age, physical condition, marital status, or professional preparation." Ironically, nursing leaders who espoused the virtues of hearth and home criticized nurses who were choosing to get married, accusing them of suddenly becoming dependent "clinging vines" in order to secure exemption from their wartime responsibility.

While the dominant traditional female roles remained that of wife and mother, nursing leaders counted on nurses to suspend those expectations while their services were needed for the war effort. To focus only on one's personal domestic responsibilities invited admonishment from others for being selfish; choosing to create a family was cause for dismissal from a nursing position.

Eventually, to solve the issue of marriage, most nursing schools discarded restrictions against married women, allowing them to enroll in classes. Also, before the year ended, the War Department allowed married nurses under forty without minors or with dependents over 14 years old to join the Army Nurse Corps. Nurses in this group were certainly shown no favoritism as the Army stipulated that they would be offered commissions only if they accepted assignments unreservedly.

Recruiters recognized that their expectations exceeded normal limits and called the phenomenon "the paradox of doing more and more with less and less." Recruiters also expected nurses to volunteer for military service regardless of the shortages they would experience in food, quinine and other medicines, supplies, equipment, appropriate uniforms, and pay. Recruitment rhetoric minimized these problems and encouraged more nurses to go to war. Editorials and articles in nursing publications were more candid and carried a tone of caution to their readers: *do not expect a short war or speedy victory*.

In hopes of stimulating recruitment activity, the National Nursing Council implemented a program it called a survey but was really a tool to establish eligibility status. The Council launched the National Survey of Graduate Nurses on New Year's Day, expecting to reach every graduate registered nurse in the nation regardless of marital status or involvement in the profession. The Council developed the survey instrument so that nurses could "let their government know of her willingness to serve either in the armed forces or as a civilian." After receiving a completed survey instrument, the Council could target each individual by mail and tailor subsequent notices to the respondent's particular category of eligibility. Throughout the year, the Council published and circulated:

- Bulletins (e.g. "Nursing Education in Wartime")

- Guides (e.g. "Distribution of Nursing Services During the War")

- Pamphlets (e.g. "Nurses to the Colors" and "Priorities for Nurses")

In addition to the written pieces, the Council used radio and other media to carry the message that more nurses were desperately needed in the military.

The American Red Cross improved its initial recruitment program as the U.S. settled into its first full year of war. For more expedient handling of applications, the Red Cross established recruitment centers in cities with a population of 25,000 or more and placed more emphasis in their advertising on recruiting for the military reserve corps - not the Red Cross itself. The Red Cross had learned that many nurses did not understand the relationship between the American Red Cross and the Army Nurse Corps. Two different groups existed within the Army Nurse Corps - the Regular Army and the Reservists. A nurse could apply directly to the Army Nurse Corps and become regular Army or go through the Red Cross Nursing Service and become a reservist. The ARC used the distinction to show that they were actually recruiting for the military not just the Red Cross.

By autumn 1944, the Army removed the responsibility for recruitment from the Red Cross. The Army itself began calling for more nurses and in an attempt to increase interest in volunteering for military service, the Army designated September 3 through September 9 as "Army Nurse Week." The Army hoped this campaign would attract one-third of the 28,900 graduates from the class of 1944, (about 9500 nurses) to military service.

Although 50,000 nurses were serving with the armed forces in December 1944, military leaders wanted to increase personnel to cover positions at additional installations around the world. The Army, like the nursing recruiters, relied heavily upon guilt to motivate nurses to volunteer for military service. One editorial expressed the Army's desperate approach:

*The Army has not enough nurses... the lives
of men, American men, are dependent upon
prompt and efficient care. Why do the Army
and Navy have to beg for nurses? There can
be only one possible reason. Nurses have not
understood the need...*

*The Surgeon General knows that without
nurses, he will be responsible to the people
of this country for unnecessary loss of life.*

The War Department perceived the nursing shortage
to be so critical, especially after the mounting
casualties caused by the Battle of the Bulge in late
1944, that the Surgeon General of the Army urgently
demanded more and more nurses. Military planners
wanted 60,000 nurses in the ANC for fiscal year
1945 but they believed that the nursing profession
could not deliver that number solely through
volunteerism. In a display of panic, and
demonstrating the dire need of increasing the military
nursing pool, the Surgeon General responded to what
he perceived as failed voluntary recruitment. He
persuaded President Roosevelt to ask Congress for
legislation to draft nurses into the military. In his
message to Congress on January 6, 1945, Roosevelt

repeated the Surgeon General's alarm when he stated:

One of the most urgent immediate requirements of the armed forces is more nurses... The present shortage of Army nurses is reflected in undue strain on the existing forces... Since volunteering has not produced the number of nurses required, I urge that the Selective Service Act be amended to provide for the induction of nurses into the armed forces... The care and treatment given to our wounded and sick soldiers have been the best known to medical science. Those standards must be maintained at all costs. We cannot tolerate a lowering of them by failure to provide adequate nursing for the brave men who stand desperately in need of it.

These drastic measures surprised the leadership within the nursing profession. The Army provided nursing recruiters with conflicting information as they vacillated about their objectives. Before the war, planners in the War Department established the nurse-to-troop ratio at 6 nurses for every 1000 men. In 1943, they estimated a troop-strength of 8,500,000 men which indicated that 51,000 nurses would be needed. Then, the War Department reduced their troop-size estimate by a million soldiers which meant they only needed about 45,000 nurses - a difference of 6000 women. At the time of the hearings on the draft legislation, the Army announced another increase in requirements from 50,000 to 70,000 nurses. This increase was known only to the Surgeon General and the President of the United States - not to the nursing profession.

Commenting on the proposed draft legislation before the State Military Affairs Committee, Katherine J. Densford, President of the American Nurse Association, voiced the views of the ANA and its members. She informed Congress that all quotas had been met in previous years, including 1944, despite the quotas being first raised, then lowered, then raised again. In December, 1943, when the Army told P&AS they needed a total of only 40,000 nurses in the Nurse Corps, the profession responded by securing that number by April of the next year, while many more qualified applicants were being turned away by the Army. News traveled quickly through the grapevine about the restrictions and many qualified nurses ceased to be interested in military service. Before the month was out, however, the Army informed P&AS that they needed a total of 50,000 nurses by April, 1945. This number was increased again to 70,000 during the Hearings. In her address before Congress during the Draft Legislation Hearings, Densford stated:

> *There is a limit beyond which nurses cannot be mobilized under any plan. This is particularly true because the duties of nurses in this wartime emergency have been extended far beyond their recognized field, in fact, they have become the "shock absorbers" for any and all unmet needs, in both military and civilian hospitals...*

Officially, the ANA accepted the draft of nurses ONLY as a first step in a draft of all women since the Women's Army Corps [WAC] and other female services had not reached their authorized strength either. Nevertheless, this bit of legislative flurry allowed nursing leaders a public voice on their own behalf during the hearings held by the House Committee on Military Affairs and the Senate

Committee on Military Affairs. The hearings proved
to some nurse leaders the tremendous importance that
their profession played in national security.

Nursing leaders believed that cranking up the
legislative vehicle to draft nurses created a problem
in recruitment because many nurses adopted a "wait-
and-see" attitude. Military leaders realized that
although volunteering increased after Pearl Harbor,
and after the invasion of North Africa almost a year
later, volunteer rates began to decrease by the
summer of 1944 as an optimistic response to news
reports detailing a successful landing at Normandy,
improved conditions in the Pacific, and perhaps an
early end to war.

Recruiters found the process of recruitment
problematic because the Army requirements for
nurses fluctuated at a crucial period of the war -
without explanations. The process of recruitment
was very complex and required clearance by the
P&AS, certification by the American Red Cross, and
commissioning by the Army Nurse Corps. The
National Nursing Council's funding for a
comprehensive public relations program was not
commensurate with its importance and expectations.

Also, the civilian sector, including hospital administrators, placed demands on women creating unwillingness within institutions to concede priorities to the military. The absence of consistently firm figures from the War Department created confusion of whether or not quotas were being met. The fluctuations of Army requirements had a catastrophic influence on enrollment and created extra work for everyone from that time until Victory in Europe Day.

Late in the war, an occasional article irresponsibly reported that nurses were not fulfilling their duty by volunteering. As large numbers of sick and wounded men entered hospitals on the homefront from all theaters of war, hospitals became grossly understaffed and civilian nurses who remained at home felt they were most needed stateside. According to Roberts, about 30,000 wounded soldiers were returning to stateside hospitals each month. The media announced that eleven hospitals had been deployed overseas without nurses. The news profoundly affected the professionally minded nurses who felt like unsubstantiated references to their unavailability was a black mark against their participation in the war effort and would restrict their struggle to professionalize. After the war ended, the truth of this incident surfaced. Military facilities needed only the "equipment" of the hospital that was sent, not personnel. As a result of these developments, however, public opinion reflected a trend in increasing negative attitudes toward the important part nurses played in the war. Nursing leaders became concerned that the prestige of the profession for which they were working had been dealt a blow. Consensus within the nursing leadership considered the draft legislation as an affront to a profession that already responded valiantly.

As the nursing profession worked to supply the military with ample medical personnel, another problem arose in recruitment and centered on the War Department's reneging on promised federal funds and personnel necessary for increasing

74

voluntary recruitment. Four thousand appointed federal recruitment officers supported WAC recruitment, but only 32 appointments worked for the Army Nursing Corps. The public relations staff was practically nonexistent, and without a publicity campaign, neither the Army Nurse Corps nor the nursing profession could influence opinion and stimulate the action needed to increase enrollment. Not until December 1944 did the War Advertising Council, working under the Office of War Information, begin an active campaign to recruit nurses. Advertising experts worked with members of the Army Nurse Corps and the American Red Cross to emphasize, display and repeat the message that the Army needed more nurses. Afterwards, the Ad Council claimed a substantial share of credit for getting nurses to respond to the Army's needs. The Ad Council secured an estimated value of donated advertising space and radio time exceeding $25,000,000 from national advertisers such as Ford Motors, Dow Chemical Company, Canada Dry, General Foods, Andrew Jergens, International Silver, W.K. Kellogg, Metropolitan Life, Prudential Life, Revlon Products, and U.S. Steel.

The Red Cross strained its resources to process recruits late in the war until the War Department issued a much welcomed order to accept all nurses who volunteered and were qualified, without regard to P&AS classifications. Also, the Army changed an important processing procedure allowing the Army Nurse Corp to accept nurses as they became available rather than on designated dates and consequently broke a chronic "bottleneck".

Of all nurses eligible for military service, one out of three volunteered and one out of four served their country in the military. Ultimately, the American Red Cross certified 103,869 nurses as eligible for military duty, of whom the Army commissioned 70,466 in their Nurse Corps.

Nursing leaders generally believed that the quota set during the draft hearings could have been met without a draft since the American Red Cross maintained a surplus of nurses in the First Reserve waiting for assignments throughout the war.

As of May 1945:

> - 47,500 nurses held a commission in the
>   Army Nurse Corps
>
> - An additional 4,500 nurses in the First
>   Reserve were awaiting assignments
>
> - At least 2,000 black nurses held credentials
>   that made them eligible for a commission in
>   the Army Nurse Corps
>
> - Approximately 2,000 eligible male nurses
>   were being ignored.

The remaining nurses could have been drawn from a pool of 42,980 active nurses who had already been classified 1-A by the Nursing Division of the Procurement and Assignment Service. With adequate funding and personnel, members of this group could have been contacted and persuaded to volunteer for military service. On May 30, 1945, however, after the Allies won victory in Europe *[V-E Day was May 8, 1945 and V-J Day was September 2, 1945]* the Surgeon General determined that the military no longer needed additional nurses for the Army Nurse Corps. Consequently, the issue of drafting the nurses lost its significance and the Senate chose not to act further on the bill.

• ✣ ⟩⟩⟩ ⟨ •

Over one hundred thousand nurses willingly volunteered their services to their country and over seventy thousand nurses were assigned to the Army Nurse Corp upon fulfilling eligibility requirements. As the United States needed women to replace manpower in the factories at home, it also needed nurses near the battlefields to reduce the loss of manpower there. Even though the federal government desperately needed women in their fight for victory, it proposed the draft for nurses only as a threat of punishment for what was perceived as a refusal do one's patriotic duty. Instead, policy-makers expected women to volunteer freely their skills and services.

Unable to trust that women would volunteer totally on their own volition, recruitment strategy relied on something stronger than legislation to elicit action - compulsion through guilt. Propaganda that surfaced in popular media, and in other tools of

78

persuasion used to sway public opinion and direct action appealed to nurses as a gender with second class status rather than adults with sharply honed scientific skills.

Nurses understood the importance of offering those skills to their nation in need while the government emphasized and exploited only nursing's orientation toward "duty and calling." As nursing leaders worked throughout the duration of the war recruiting nurses for military service, responsibility for service and action at the battlefront fell to the rank-and-file nurses who actually went to war and cared for combatants. Recruiters at home expected nurses who were going overseas to arise to "the challenge" in the same spirit as their colleagues at Pearl Harbor, Bataan, and Corregidor who had faced enemy attack and who lifted their profession to "a place of honor in national esteem." As I will demonstrate in the next chapter, nurses fulfilled these expectations placed on them and met the demands of war with courage and grace.

Chapter Three

At the Front Lines:
Expectations and Realities
of the War Experience

Nurses who volunteered for the Army Nurse Corps during World War II entered as officers with a commission equal to that of at least a Second Lieutenant. As an elite and important segment of the military, nurses had the right to expect the Army to prepare them for battlefield conditions under which they would perform their duties. But when the United States deployed its first troops to the war front, including nursing units, the Army had not invested in preparation programs for the nurses. The Army also neglected to provide nurses with appropriate clothing and adequate equipment. Fortunately, in terms of behavior, conduct and nursing ability, nursing customs carried over into the Army.

The rigorous and disciplined training that nurses received in school assisted them in dealing with the hardships they encountered overseas as they relied on their traditions of stoicism, self-sacrifice and devotion to duty. Nurses who published accounts of their often brutal experiences in autobiographies and in professional journals generally described their ordeals in a positive manner, however, minimizing the hardships they endured. And even though nurses endured severe hardships, they maintained high morale among themselves comparable to, or even better than, the typical enlisted soldier. Unlike the nurses, enlisted men received physical training, appropriate equipment and uniforms, and rest periods between military campaigns.

As the war unfolded, the War Department eventually developed training programs and produced appropriate clothing for the Army Nurse Corps. Ultimately, the wartime experience and performance of the Army Nurse Corps served to create an environment in which individual nurses gained confidence in their abilities and the desire to work toward improving their workplace conditions.

Even though Army nurses had received advanced education and assumed extensive responsibilities, their commissions at the beginning of the war were only "relative." Relative rank meant nurses did not enjoy the same privileges of authority as other military women and men of the same rank and grade. Also, under relative rank status, although nurses' pay rates were nearly equitable with other officers', they were not entitled to dependent benefits or other allowances.

Military strategy called for nurses to accompany combatants overseas, but the Army provided no basic training programs early in the war for nurses in the military. Perhaps one explanation of the Army's failure to prepare women for war is that the men directing America's war plans wanted to perpetuate the illusion that military service would not place nurses in danger. In other words, if nurses were required to undergo preparations to deal with dangers, they might assume they would be working under perilous conditions and refuse to volunteer. This line of reasoning proved to be false, however, since nurses held a realistic view about the conditions they would encounter and responded favorably to training when it became available.

Before the Army developed formal training for the nurse corps, the chief nurse or commanding officer occasionally developed limited impromptu training regimens. These exercises occupied recruits' free time during long waiting periods before reaching their destinations. One chief nurse stationed in North Africa decided that her newly arrived unit of nurses should learn to march as they waited for their initial shipment of supplies. One nurse remembered, "Oh, it was so hot on that march but then a couple of trucks came by and we hopped on for a ride back to camp. She never made us march again."

To instruct nurses in more appropriate and applicable skills, the Army finally established the first basic training center in the autumn of 1943 for Army Nurses. The fledgling training center at Fort Devens, Massachusetts prepared new ANC members in the "Army Way" of nursing. Subsequently, two other centers opened at Fort Sam Houston, Texas and Camp McCoy, Wisconsin. The four-week training period covered 192 hours of instruction that included ward management, nursing procedures, transportation and care of the wounded, military courtesy and correspondence, and the organizational structure of the Army and the Army Nurse Corps. Five full-time faculty members, including three Army nurses and two medical administrative officers, taught all of the courses. Special guest lecturers were invited to teach various courses as well. In addition to classroom instruction, the trainees received practical training in drills, bivouac and calisthenics.

Nurses enthusiastically agreed that the training program helped them make necessary adjustments from civilian to military life and provided them with a feeling of confidence in their abilities. To make the training program appear more palatable, reports written by observers at the training centers emphasized the sport and recreational nature of the maneuvers. One nurse even claimed the obstacle course was "fun." After completing the course and mastering the physical skills, this nurse and her colleagues grew more confident in their survival capabilities and felt "quite ready and even anxious to go anywhere and do what is expected of us to the greatest of our ability."

During basic training, nurses learned useful skills applicable to a wartime setting. They learned to improvise treatment with objects readily available in the field. Nurses learned to make bedpans out of newspapers, bed cradles out of barrel staves, and stretchers from trousers. Instructors utilized training films and flash cards, and offered young nurses valuable advice on "how to handle any soldier with a firm and gentle hand," emphasizing the importance of "motherly" qualities. When the nurses completed the training course, they were convinced that "the soldier is the most important person in the world."

Before the end of the war, basic training became a mandatory and practical prelude to the nurses' tour of duty. Nurses greatly benefited from this valuable program in which they "lived like soldiers, dressed like soldiers... and like good solders, learned to obey commands." When they completed the course, the basic training graduates had gained knowledge, confidence, independence and pride. As they walked across the gangway onto the troop ships carrying them to battlefronts across the globe, these nurses now "walked with a purpose."

Within 48 hours of notification, the Army expected its overseas-bound nurses to proceed to the designated port of embarkation. Each nurse took her oath of office before beginning the trip and she carried her orders and official papers on her person if traveling alone (the chief nurse carried all papers when the nurses traveled in a group). The orders instructed the nurse to guard her conversations while in transit, and to be careful not to reveal information related to her service or destination. Usually the final destination was kept secret by the War Department and revealed only after the ship had left its harbor. Nurses typically traveled by train to reach the place of departure but if time was limited they were allowed priority status on commercial airplane flights. Like all officers, each nurse assumed personal responsibility for travel expenses to the port, and then the Army reimbursed her at $4.00 per day upon completion of the journey.

While undergoing the processing procedure at the port, nurses roomed at nearby camps or received billets in local hotels where they might stay from 48 hours to two weeks waiting to ship out. Processing included a final physical examination, an update of immunizations and vaccines, and certification of blood type. Each nurse then received metal identification tags with her vital information engraved on it. Many nurses found the final processing period to be their first opportunity since volunteering to ask military-related questions.

Unlike enlisted personnel who were issued all essential items required for overseas duty including duffle bags for carrying their gear, the Army expected each nurse to acquire carrying cases at her own expense. She needed a footlocker [B-Bag] for storing the bulk of her possessions and a carry-on suitcase [A-Bag] for keeping items she needed accessible while traveling. To save precious cargo space, nurses could take only essential personal items and articles of clothing on their journey. The Army considered decorative objects excess baggage, but many nurses chose to include some beloved mementos in their possessions.

During the processing time, nurses learned to pack their "A-Bags" and "B-Bags" efficiently. This was important because B-Bags and other heavy luggage that would be stored in the hold of the ship while en route to the battlefront and therefore not available until reaching the final destination.

Deploying nurses also received a crash course in equipment use and censorship policies. Nurses spent their last few days in the States searching for any last-minute articles they would possibly need for the next two or three years. They made out wills and filled out the paper work to have their pay sent home. At last, when the alert came and instructions for departure were posted, each nurse completed a "safety arrival card" addressed to her nearest relative which would be released after the port received notice of a safe arrival.

Dressed in full uniform, carrying helmets, gas masks, field bags and canteens, the departing nurses "marched determinedly across the gangplank; and when on deck, they turned towards shore and rendered a smart parting salute."

Nurses endured varying experiences during their voyages to the war front. Theresa Archard left for overseas duty in August, 1942. She traveled as part of a "formidable convoy" that was in transit to Scotland for eleven days. To while away the hours on board the ship, men and women played card games, played musical instruments, performed calisthenics, sang, read, played Lexicon in the lounge, formed friendships and developed romances.

Dorothy Chinnis left in a ship convoy from Camp Gilma, New Jersey with the 58th Station Hospital from Fort Jackson, South Carolina, bound for North Africa. The trip took fourteen days and only when the ship reached the Rock of Gibraltar did her unit learn of their mission and destination. On the trip over, Chinnis recalled, "The boat was crowded and the water was rough... and even now, I don't care much for an afternoon on the water." But another nurse described her ocean voyage as a pleasant and enjoyable travel experience and the harbor of her destination "equally as beautiful as the one I had said farewell to."

For many nurses, reaching their destinations became the first experiences of the hardships of war as they confronted the organizational demands of military life. A year after Pearl Harbor, the official uniform allowance for each nurse included the following:

Item	Allowance
Cape, blue wool	1
Caps, blue field	1
Caps, white cotton	6
Coat, blue wool	1
Gloves, black kid	1 pair
Gloves, blue wool	1 pair
Insignia, A.N.C.	4
Insignia, U.S.	3
Muffler, blue wool	1
Overcoat, blue wool w/ removable lining	1
Overshoes	1 pair
Shoes, black	2 pairs
Shoes, white	2 pairs
Skirt, blue wool	1
Sweater, blue wool	1
Tie, black	1
Uniforms, blue cotton	6
Uniforms, white cotton	6
Waists, blue cotton	2
Waists, white cotton	2

Not included in the official list of uniform items were slacks and durable footwear - two items that make physically demanding work less problematic. Even though the Army did not issue regulation slacks or boots at this time, it did suggest that "for the voyage, two pairs of dark blue slacks, one of wool and one of a washable fabric, and two dark blue slipover sweaters" could be purchased at the nurses' personal expense. Additional field equipment issued by the Army to nurses might include bed rolls, mattress covers, blankets, tents, tent poles, tent pins, helmets, gas masks, canvas field bags, mess gear, pistol belts, first aid kits, and canteens. It's possible that the Army's reluctance to issue trousers to nurses reflected contemporary conventions that women typically did not wear them outside the home. In fact, Greta Garbo and Marlene Dietrich made headlines when, to the amazement of their fans, they appeared so-dressed in public.

Since the Army did not advocate wearing a more practical uniform, nursing units entered the North African campaign early in the war ill-clothed for their assignment. Some nurses in the first wave of the North African invasion reported that they waded ashore in their skirted uniforms. The chief nurse of one unit docking in North Africa ordered her nurses to disembark in full uniform (which at that time still consisted of the navy blue skirt and jacket), while carrying gas masks and an impregnated clothing kit. The kit included special clothing treated with protective chemicals to repel the effects of gas warfare, but would have been difficult to don over a skirted suit.

Nurses suffered other incidents of being unsuitably prepared because of the Army's oversight. To keep warm in the cold and rainy seasons, nurses assumed responsibility for locating and purchasing, at their own expense, men's G.I. long woolen underwear, men's coveralls and field jackets, men's fatigue hats and men's G.I. boots at the Post Exchange (PX). Then, when the nurses' superiors ordered them to climb aboard the 2-ton trucks for transportation to the next camp, they could scale tailgates, scramble across cargo and move and stretch in relative comfort and modesty.

Military officials emphasized the feminine nature of the nursing staff and its contribution to lifting the lonely soldier's morale overseas. In the meantime, officials overlooked women's particular needs. Whereas the PX generally maintained a generous stock of men's clothing, nurses found it difficult to locate and purchase stockings, panties, bras, pajamas, and other female garments in the PX. It was also difficult to purchase hair pins, feminine napkins and other feminine health care products.

Even though the Army Nurse Corps expected each nurse to take care of herself in the field, including hiking across rough terrain, the Army initially issued children's shoes with a top sewn on to them to nurses rather than practical hiking boots. According to one nurse, "they were not comfortable for walking long distances but they felt good when walking on paths covered with large gravel."

Eventually, to meet the special needs of the Army nurses in combat, the Army engaged Dorothy Shaver, Vice-President of Lord and Taylor of New York City, to design new women's uniforms for the Quartermaster General. Shaver's designers interviewed nurses who had served in the Philippines, soliciting their opinions and preferences on special features of serviceability and appearance. Shaver made the new uniforms from olive drab, replacing the navy blue. The new uniform became a smart ensemble that paralleled that of the Army officer. According to official reports in *The American Journal of Nursing*, Shaver's uniforms were "attractive on various types of figures, comfortable to work in, and useful in all conditions and all climates... ."

For rugged terrain, the Army issued nurses a special heavy cotton herringbone twill work suit with trousers cut in women's sizes, and high field shoes made on women's shoe-lasts and designed to fit a woman's foot. The Army planned to issue these new uniforms to nurses overseas by July 1, 1943. Many nurses continued to improvise on their personal uniforms until the end of the war.

When a hospital unit reached its destination in the field, a detail unit set up the transient tent city where nurses lived under the same conditions as soldiers.

They had access to neither heat for their tents nor hot water for bathing. Light for reading and other personal activities came from candles, lanterns or flashlights. Groups of four to six nurses slept in tents sparsely furnished with bedrolls and folding cots, and like soldiers, nurses stood in line for everything from meals to washing. Nurses remained exhausted much of the time - working twelve-hour shifts and even longer at times. Bending over the rows and rows of cots barely eighteen inches from the ground fatigued their backs as did slogging through the mud between tents.

Nevertheless, nurses continued to work in spite of the hardships. They knew that their greatest contribution to defense would be to minimize the loss of lives. The medical team worked from the assumption that "every war-torn human must be salvaged." To achieve this aim, hospitals maintained close proximity to the battlefield. Field hospitals followed closely behind attack lines moving in tandem with the combat units. Each field hospital generally employed 22 officers, 18 nurses, and 190 enlisted men divided into three hospitalization units (receiving, treating, and evacuating) and a headquarters section. Typically, patients stayed in the field hospital for only two or three days. When they could withstand travel, the patients were sent back to the evacuation hospitals.

A little further back from the battlefield than the field hospitals, were the evacuation hospitals (EVACs) and auxiliary surgical groups. The auxiliary surgical groups consisted of a team of highly skilled surgeons, trained technicians, and surgical nurses. This group worked as independent units with the evacuation hospitals inside the combat zone and "leap-frogged" one another on the battlefield. The surgical group carried everything it needed to function, making it very mobile and versatile. The auxiliary surgical group treated the most urgent and non-transportable cases until they could be evacuated to the rear. Saving a wounded soldier's life required three crucial steps:

1. Quick transportation
2. Early medical attention
3. Professional nursing care.

Nurses took the third step seriously. In any given night, nurses may have assisted with major surgery or even performed minor surgical procedures themselves. Procedures such as removing shell fragments, setting broken bones, amputating or reconstructing badly damaged limbs and tissue - all of which may have taken place during air raids.

The Army needed highly trained nurses because medical care was given under extreme tension and pressure. One nurse, commenting about working under the pressures of battlefront conditions said, "there is no time to teach a helper, no time to tell anyone else where to find things."

Nurses realized the unique importance of their function and were aware that only essential personnel accompanied the invading forces as they crossed into enemy territory and that each person must perform his or her own part proficiently. The medical unit was a self sufficient organization, reduced to a minimum, "and each worker a jack-of-all-trades."

Those "jacks" or *"jills"* rather, adeptly modified, improvised and substituted their equipment and supplies when the normal equipment could not be obtained. Nurses' fundamental knowledge, skills and experience in the basic principles of nursing care provided them with the means to adapt to new and novel situations. Their sense of professionalism helped nurses "remain calm in the midst of confusion, quiet nerves in a tent shaken by exploding shells, [and use] intelligent responses to a rising tide of emergencies." As nurses found they could stand the test of performing under difficult conditions and their confidence grew in themselves, they began to believe that even though many women could learn to march long distances and crawl on their bellies under fire, only "nurses" offered countless life-saving skills along with the cool demeanor required in a crisis situation.

In addition to managing their medical duties, nurses dealt with personal threats of war as they suffered individual tragedies. Nurses fell ill, were taken prisoner, were declared missing in action, and were killed or wounded in action. A total of 201 Army nurses lost their lives during World War II, some of whom drowned when their ships were torpedoed while traveling in military convoys. Six Army nurses drowned when their vessel, the U.S. Hospital Ship "Comfort", was sunk by enemy attack on April 28, 1945. Nurses accompanied invasion parties that landed under fire on beachheads. Aerial bombings killed nurses on duty in hospital units barely behind the front lines.

Nurses stationed in Hawaii and the Philippines were the first to confront battlefield conditions when the Japanese attacked the islands in December 1941. Sixty-six nurses stationed in the Philippines remained prisoners of the Japanese from May 1942 until their liberation 37 months later. In Europe, enemy troops captured Lieutenant Reba Z. Whittle of the 813th Medical Air Evacuation Transport Squadron after Germans shot her plane down during a medical evacuation mission over Aachen, Germany. Thirteen nurses were listed as missing in action when their plane crash-landed in Albania on November 8, 1943. Underground partisans helped them escape Nazi-held territory after more than six weeks behind German lines. Second Lieutenant Ruth M. Gardiner was the first World War II Army Nurse to be killed in a theater of operations when her plane crashed during an air evacuation mission.

For other nurses, battlefront conditions began during the Allied invasion of North Africa after the United States officially entered the war. This strategy was part of the Allied plan to liberate the Mediterranean coast of Africa from German occupation. On the second night after arrival in North Africa, Dorothy Chinnis experienced her first air raid. She recalled watching briefly the sparks and the fantastic light show, then hearing the sounds that followed. "I thought the world was coming to an end, I couldn't have imagined beforehand what it would be like." Disregarding the Red Cross signs plainly painted on the hospital buildings where Chinnis worked, German bombers pelted the area frequently with bombs, destroying water systems and buildings. Ironically, the German POWs working in some of the Allied hospitals often felt protective toward the nurses and attempted to shield them from falling debris when possible.

After the close calls Chinnis experienced from the German bombings, she was not afraid of being shot, for she never thought she would live long enough to confront enemy troops. In fact, taking Atabrine frightened Chinnis more than the prospects of being shot. This medicine was given to prevent malaria but it made her and many other nurses "deathly sick" until a physician told her to "forget those pills until you can get something on your stomach."

Fires were not allowed in camp during this time for cooking or for warmth, and the only food available was cold C-rations - except on one occasion. One night, the cook managed to serve a particularly aromatic stew and someone asked where "that old lumpy camel had gotten to." The cook remained silent on the source of the meat, but after hearing the reference, Chinnis was unable to eat her share of the meal and continued to survive on the cheese, peanut butter and bread that were standard fare until food shipments became available.

Following months in the field without proper diet and rest, many nurses fell ill along with some of the enlisted men and doctors. Archard contracted malaria and the deadening fatigue that accompanied it. She needed rest but saw no hope of it in the near future. She lost over twenty-five pounds and her skin took on a color "yellow as a duck's foot." Her hair, which had once been thick, brown and curly, became thin and grey. She and the other nurses needed fresh milk, vegetables, and vitamins but her unit did not have consistent access to basic supplies. After twenty months away from home, Archard was finally sent stateside to recuperate at Stark General Hospital in Charleston, South Carolina.

Medical units seldom worked under less than crisis conditions, but when a lull in battlefield casualties did occur, nurses spent their spare time sight-seeing or frequenting the Red Cross Nurses' Club. At the club, they could purchase ice cream and other treats unavailable at camp. Having a few hours of recreation in order to leave worries and cares temporarily behind broke up the nurses' routine a little and helped lift their morale. Other forms of recreation included informal baseball and volleyball games between enlisted men and the male officers. Sometimes volunteers staged plays or pageants for the unit's entertainment. Movies were available for viewing in the mess tents, sometimes twice a week. While stationed in North Africa, Chinnis cites no fewer than 31 movies in her diary, including films like 'Pride of the Yankees', 'The Great Mister Gildersleeve', 'Suspicion', 'Intermezzo', 'Andy Hardy's Double Life', 'God's Little Acre' and 'Juarez', among others. And on occasions, USO entertainers like Bob Hope passed through the area.

Receiving mail and packages remained a constant morale-builder for nurses. Friends and relatives at home found that some of the most useful items to send to the nurse in foreign service were hosiery, cosmetics, toothbrushes, tissues, and soap. These items were difficult to find overseas as were hair pins, curlers, shoe polish, rustproof safety pins, garters, sanitary belts and pads, and sewing kits. Other scarce items coveted by the nurses overseas included fountain pens and ink, writing paper, flashlights, games, playing cards, non-electric flatirons, and coffee pots. Postal restrictions allowed packages that weighed no more than 11 pounds, and they had to be within stated dimensions. The Army Postal Service requested that food *not* be sent overseas and only one package per person be mailed each week. These regulations were very often ignored by stateside friends and families. Written correspondence did not have as many restrictions, and for a quick, secure, and inexpensive way to send correspondence, many people relied on 'V-Mail'. V-mail was an efficient mail system initiated by the U.S. Postal Service to reduce the size and bulk of correspondence between military men and women in service abroad and their loved ones at home. Each piece was a letter and envelope combination. The letter-writer wrote on one side of the sheet in the prescribed area, then folded the sheet and addressed the outer portion to the recipient. This letter was then photographed and reduced to thumbnail size onto microfilm. The microfilm took up a fraction of the space that the normal size mail would need, saving precious cargo room for food and other necessary provisions shipped overseas. The microfilm was sent on to a special receiving area near the addressee where each letter was printed and delivered to the receiver.

Army nurses cherished receiving news reports and updates as often as possible. Even bad news was better than no news since lack of information created more stress than not being informed. Nurses received news from the official Army newspaper *The Stars and Stripes*, word-of-mouth, or the radio. Receiving news through official channels was not a timely way to get information. In fact, Chinnis heard about President Roosevelt's death from the Mayor of Mericourt (a small town in France near the hospital where she was posted) before the base received official word of his death. Postal restrictions prevented families from sending local newspapers overseas and letters with news typically arrived eight to twelve days after posting. Often, local citizens were more informed than the Americans, and nurses frequently heard about world events in the local shops more quickly than through official channels.

Friendship remained a powerful coping mechanism for confronting the demands of war. When morale in Chinnis' unit dropped, the nurses took solace in each other's company. She recalled that "we were all in it together. It was helpful to have each other over there, to cry on each other's shoulders". A feeling of group identity or camaraderie developed and emerged among the women just as it emerged among men in their various units. A "mysterious pride in one's own platoon" stated one nurse, "offers us very real comfort and security in being in the same hot water with fellows of exact status".

Yet, although male leadership encouraged camaraderie among the male soldiers, it did not consistently promote camaraderie among the nurses. Archard described an ordeal her outfit experienced early in the war while waiting in England for assignment:

> *The Commanding Officer decided that it*
> *Was bad for morale for nurses to become*
> *too friendly with each other and had made*
> *it a point to separate friends by placing them*
> *in different units. The bitterness that piled*
> *up after that was alarming and many tears*
> *were shed...*

*It's bad enough being in a strange country
without taking your friends away from you....
How did he know which of us were friends?
He didn't know any of us, and he hasn't
spoken two words to most of us.*

Nevertheless, friendship alone could not prevent some mental breakdowns. Archard reported that there were two cases of nurses breaking down with "hysterics - they could stand no more". When battle casualties began to flow into the hospitals, there was little time for rest or diversions away from the bloodshed. Archard wondered:

*...why can't we get away for a week or two,
away from those horrible mangled bodies,
just rest a little and forget sickness? An
army could rest before going into a battle,
but a hospital couldn't.*

One young nurse wrote home:

*It is now 3 A.M. Most of my patients are
asleep so I have a chance to write a few
words... Oh, aunt, I feel so tired lately,
my stomach feels to be upside down.
When I am asleep I wake up constantly
and can't get a rest... Recently we are*

110

*getting very bad casualties. It makes
me shiver to just look at them. You
can't imagine, aunt, what we see over
here. I will never forget it - it is heart-
breaking.*

*One of my patients, only 24, has a piece
of shrapnel in his heart, another 29 and
married, has both legs off - his hips are
broken, his intestines exposed. Another,
19, was shot through the abdomen, and
after the Germans found him lying, they
kicked him and shot him into the head,
to finish him... . He suffers much. His
eyes are gone. I have also two patients
who were shot through the brain. They
lost their eyesight and are crazy. This
is just a part of what we see.*

After working under battlefront conditions for
sustained amounts of time, tempers flared, and many
nurses became curt and irritated with each other.
One strategy for dealing with short tempers was to
avoid each other when possible to prevent "friction
and clashing of personalities." Even under these
extreme conditions, nurses strove to maintain the
professionalism they learned during their nursing
education.

In addition to civilian nursing ethics and principles, nurses internalized Army Nurse Corps conventions. Corps expectations included:

> *...duty well performed, honor in all things, readiness to accept increased responsibility, a meticulous appearance at all times, the loyalty of all from the highest to the lowest and observation of social amenities.*

The most significant core value remained 'courtesy'. A high-ranking officer in the Army Nurse Corp described *courtesy* as "acts of politeness, of civility and of respect, and includes a full and proper appreciation for the rights of others." Additionally, this officer stressed that an Army nurse should never "bring discredit upon her uniform by word or action. She should not volunteer excuses unless an explanation is requested, and she should not convey gossip, slander, harsh criticism and faulting." Perhaps the most important code of the Army Nurse Corps was to never go over the head of the chief nurse.

Nurses posed few discipline problems in the Army Nurse Corps. They came to the Corps pre-disciplined from their civilian nursing training. As one observer noted:

> *The rookie of the Army Nurse Corps*
> *comes into the Army a thoroughly*
> *disciplined person. She must be a*
> *registered nurse, which means that*
> *she has been subjected to the rigid*
> *discipline of the nursing profession*
> *over a period of years. She has*
> *learned to put her own comfort and*
> *convenience second to the job in hand,*
> *as a matter of course. She is used to*
> *taking orders, and she takes them in*
> *her stride, without resentment, just*
> *as she takes everything else.*

One chief nurse who was confident in her unit's abilities even though its members had not received Army training, remarked, "The fact of being a nurse connotated *[sic]* a professional type of behavior. I told the nurses what (as their chief) I expected of them and they never let me down." Chinnis believed she actually had a little more freedom in the Army Nurse Corps than during her nurse training. The discipline she learned in school carried over into the Corps with few exceptions. Chinnis saw similarities between the rules and regulations of both institutions but felt Army regulations, in addition to nursing discipline, were unnecessary. "We were sent over to do a job, to work as a team," Chinnis recalls. "And no one wanted to let the others down."

Chinnis and a majority of her fellow nurses were self-motivated, by their very calling, to do the best job they were capable of. However, a few nurses did fall short of the "angel in white" image. Chinnis recalled that on one occasion a young single pregnant nurse, who was attached to a different hospital, came through their camp on her way home. Little was said of the incident and comments that were made were sympathetic. Many nurses felt it was a miracle that similar situations were not more prevalent.

Finding instances of reprobate conduct among the nurses is incredibly difficult to uncover, especially since official nursing sources, as well as individual nurses, tend to protect one another's reputations out of a sense of professional loyalty. Nevertheless, official statistics reflect that pregnancy rates for single nurses remained lower than extramarital fertility among the general population in the states. Nurses in the Army who did become pregnant received an honorable discharge with no reference to marital status.

One might suspect overwhelming abuse of alcohol under the trying circumstances of battlefield duty. But there is little evidence to support that supposition. Chinnis recalled a couple of nurses who would drink alcohol to excess at times. "But not too much," she clarified, "we had to work too hard and they would have been weeded out if they weren't performing."

Even with an excellent reputation, controversy concerning nurses' images and roles followed them into battle. Some observers considered nurses "plain, industrious, and uncomplying" as they accompanied the troops around the globe. Some men, in their resentment toward having women attached to medical units overseas, assailed the nurses by making slurs against their physical appearance. For example, the mess officer traveling with the 38th Evacuation Hospital from Charlotte, North Carolina kept detailed accounts of his experiences. When the nurses arrived to join his outfit at Fort Bragg he wrote:

> *The nurses have moved in next door,*
> *or rather the next barracks. I have*
> *looked them over and I know Powers*
> *or Zeigfield would never have picked*
> *them out. They wear a blue denim*
> *outfit similar to the enlisted men's*
> *fatigue uniform or more like what a*
> *Negro would plow in. That doesn't*
> *help their rather forlorn appearance*
> *either. But with their coming came*
> *special orders that we must keep our*
> *shades down and not be caught out*
> *without a shirt on...*

Nurses were sent to war to offer medical services rather than to be potential sex objects for the solders. Yet Bernice Wilbur, the director of all the nurses in North Africa, boasted that "my girls managed to keep their femininity. They saw to it that their hair looked neat and attractive, and they didn't let themselves grow careless about makeup." Other nursing leaders asserted, however, that nurses do more than just lend a pretty face to an otherwise drab camp environment and attempted to portray nursing in the Army and Navy as a thoughtful process, one that involved "applications of the newest principles developed by medical science."

In addition to the role of physical healers, though, nurses nonetheless served an additional value to the armed forces in combat; that of morale-builder. In fact, morale-building was such an important role for nurses in the war that policy makers in the War Department justified placing them in extremely dangerous areas in which nurses lost their lives. For example, the evacuation hospital attached to the Fifth Army Amphibious Forces arrived on the Anzio beachhead on January 27, 1944, three days after the invasion by Allied forces. As a front line field hospital, the medical personnel cared for the most desperately injured soldiers well within the range of fire. Throughout the day on February 10, 1944, air raids remained constant; stray bombs fell and flak from anti-aircraft guns strafed the tent city. Patients urged the nurses to "go to the foxholes!" but the nurses refused to leave their charges. A direct hit in the nurses' area killed First Lieutenant Glenda Spelhaug from Crosby, North Dakota and Second Lieutenant LaVerne Farquhar from Sidney, Texas. Just three days earlier on the same beachhead

German bombs hit an evacuation hospital killing four other nurses, one of whom was a Red Cross nurse who had served as an Army Nurse in the First World War but was refused a commission in this war because of the age requirement.

Major Norman T. Kirk, Surgeon General of the U.S. Army, believed nurses' presence at the battlefield was absolutely necessary for victory. Justifying their presence under such dangerous conditions, Kirk stated:

> *I consider the sight of these American Women more important to recovery than any psychological factor in the course of their treatment... They are not only trying to heal broken bodies, but they are also trying to heal broken spirits.*

Although he had fielded complaints about sending women so far forward Kirk declared that the nurses never registered a complaint and were "always cheerful, always morale-building, never downhearted." One chief nurse explained why her nurses did not complain. "We didn't have time... we worked so long and so hard that there was no time for reflection. When we went to bed, we slept."

A surgeon of the Fifth Army, General Joseph I. Martin also defended the presence of nurses at the Anzio beachhead in a report claiming that:

> *Had the nurses been removed, the act would have betrayed to the combat troops the gravity of their own plight. Nurses certainly are not expendable, but in a situation as critical as that which developed on the beachhead - when subjective factors determined whether a line would hold or crack - the nurses assumed a major symbolic importance... The presence of the nurses on the beachhead constituted a ringing affirmation of our determination to hold what we had.*

Indeed, the presence of nurses in the hospitals overseas affected the morale of the men with whom they worked and for whom they cared. One enlisted man attached to a hospital unit wrote to his wife:

> *The nurses add a bit of color and I can see now why the Army likes to have them along. They give a touch that the men can't give. A skirt going by the cot just makes the hospital seem different. And they can write home for the patients better than the men can, they know what to say... The effect is astounding.*

The touch of femininity, the knowledge that a woman is around gives a wounded man courage and confidence and a feeling of security. And the more feminine she looks, the better.

A wounded soldier wrote the following laudatory poem:

You never see her on parade,
Like WAACs and WAVES and such;
She's much too busy working hard
To keep away Death's touch.

I won't forget her tender skill,
From Pvt. Joe to Capt. Bill;
My thanks to you! I wish folks knew
The hell you've seen and waded through;

I'd like to tell the universe;
God bless you, keep you, Army Nurse.

Although the official and primary role for nurses was that of healer, many nurses realistically filled the role of romantic partner, too. The Army established rules against fraternizing with enlisted men but nurses were free to mix socially with male officers. For example, First Lieutenant Dorothy Daley married Lieutenant Emanuel "Boots" Engel, Jr. while they were both stationed in the Philippines just before its fall to the Japanese. After the wedding, in which both bride and groom wore fatigues, the couple took a six-hour honeymoon. Subsequently Boots followed his unit to another area and was promptly listed as missing in action.

Another wartime romance involved Second Lieutenant Dorothy Chinnis who became engaged to Jack Light before she left the states, with plans to marry after the war. After spending nine months in North Africa and nine months in Italy, her unit moved north through France as the Allies pushed toward Germany. When Light's unit joined an outfit in Europe, the couple revised their wedding plans to include a ceremony in the little town of Ravenel, France on January 15, 1945 which was followed by another ceremony at the base. The couple honeymooned in liberated Paris.

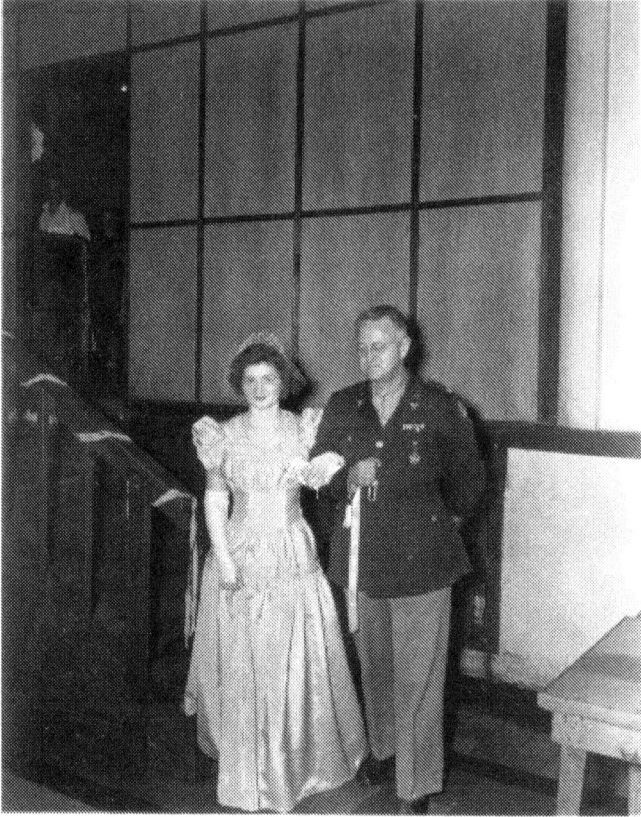

Dorothy Chinnis, on her wedding day.

Colonel Cady gave her away.

(Dorothy C. Light)

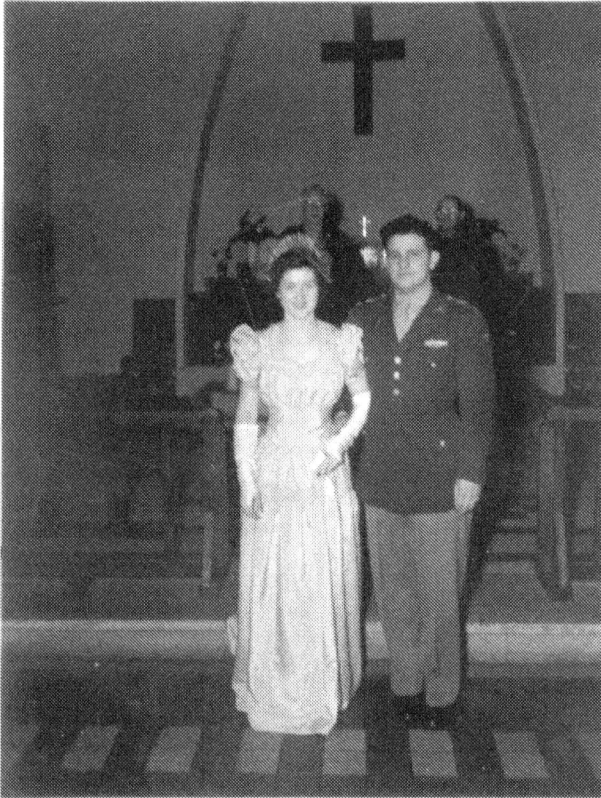

Mr. and Mrs. Jack Light

Wedding day – January 15, 1945

(Dorothy C. Light)

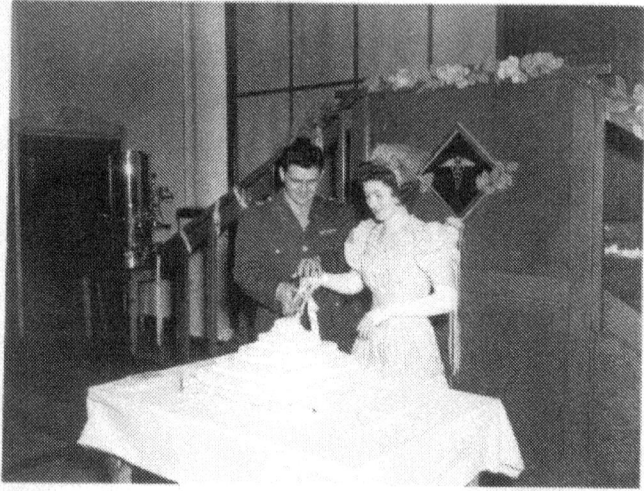

Cutting the wedding cake

(Dorothy C. Light)

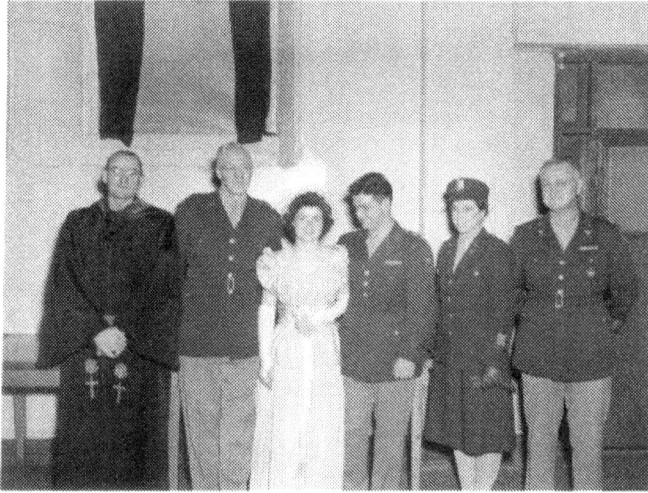

L-R: Colonel Lecrone (Light's chaplain), Chaplain Hook (Chinnis' chaplain), Dorothy Chinnis Light, Jack Light, Major Spaulding (Chinnis' chief nurse) and Colonel Cady (Head of Hospital)

(Dorothy C. Light)

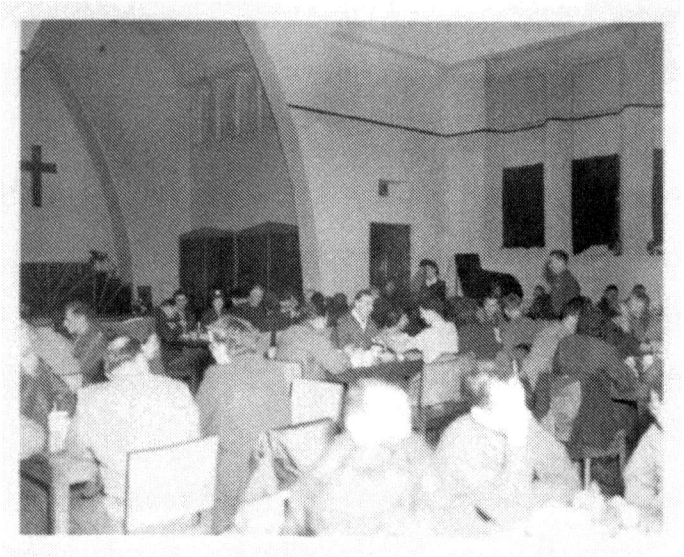

Wedding Party in the Chapel

(Dorothy C. Light)

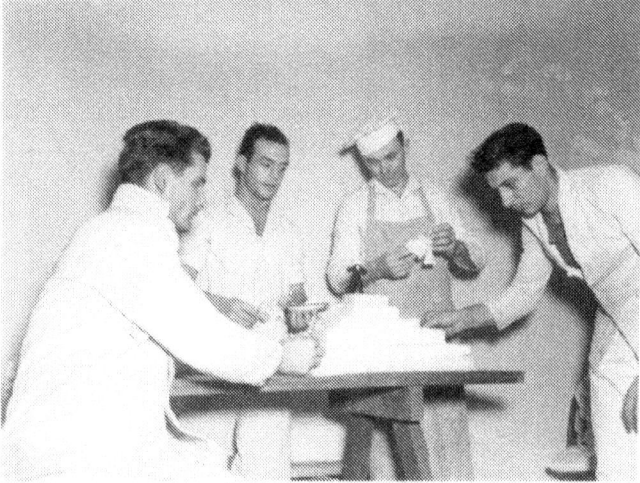

Placing finishing touches on the wedding cake

(Dorothy C. Light)

This is My Personal

DIARY

Dorothy Elizabeth Chinnis

2nd Lt. A.N.C.

Five Years
from
19 4 3 *to* 19 46

Personal diary of Dorothy Chinnis

Kept for the duration of her military service

(Dorothy C. Light)

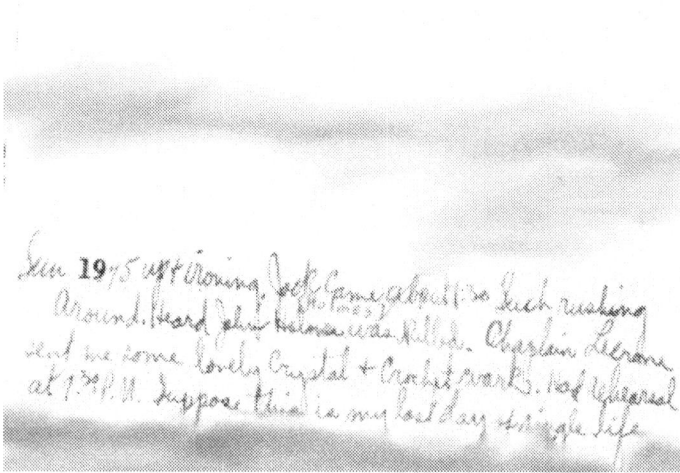

Diary entry for the day before the wedding.
Sunday, January 14, 1945

"Up and ironing. Jack came about 1:30. Such rushing around. Heard John Holmes was killed. Chaplain Lecrone sent me some lovely crystal and crochet work. Had rehearsal at 7:30pm. Suppose this is my last day of single life."

[Author's note: Holmes would have been best man]

(Dorothy C. Light)

Diary entry for the wedding day.
Monday, January 15, 1945

"*My Wedding Day*. Ready to go to the Mayor of Mericourt to be married in civil services @ 10. Jack bought me for 36 Francs. Ha! Ha! Wedding @ 3. Sgt Hosey sang. POWs played. Very nice reception @ 6. Had dinner @ Col Cady's table. Slept in Mericourt."

(Dorothy C. Light)

Diary entry for the day after the wedding.
Tuesday, January 16, 1945

*"Up & away for Paris. Jack, Dutka and I in a Jeep.
Stopped in Neuf-Chateau at a French place & warmed
with hot bricks & 3 other stops. Spent the night in Hotel of
Paris. Very nice indeed."*

(Dorothy C. Light)

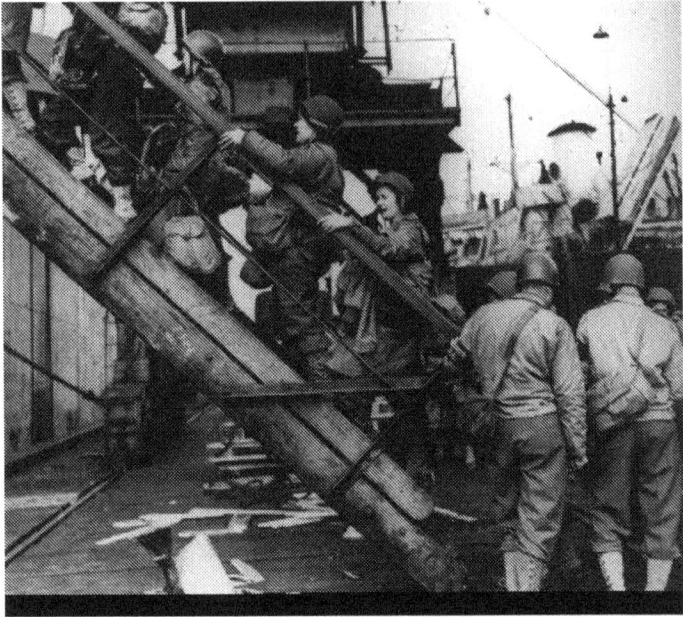

Army Nurses boarding a ship for overseas duty

(ANC/U.S. Army)

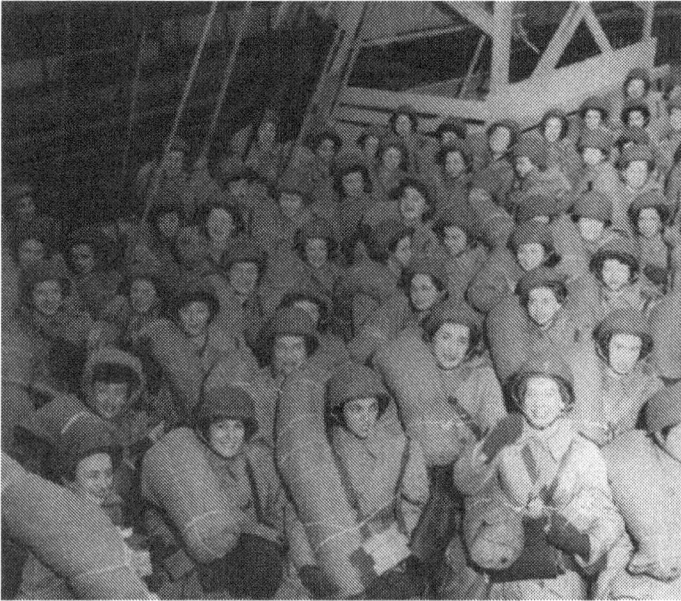

Army Nurses carrying personal gear

(ANC/U.S. Army)

Marriage to a member of the Armed Forces no longer affected an Amy Nurse's assignment to duty after early 1943. Before this policy was amended, a married nurse could be transferred to a new station if she and her husband served at the same base.

Rank-and-file nurses at battlefront confronted a variety of experiences. Although the image of the roles of nurses was a one-dimensional representation of angels-of-mercy or morale-builder, in reality, Army nurses also filled roles as administrators, planners, leaders, followers, technicians, and practitioners. Nurses brought strength, competency, bravery, and intelligence to the Army Nurse Corps. Even before the Army sought their help, the nursing profession had begun preparing for war as early as 1939. When war became a reality for America, the nurses adapted to military life despite the Army's failure to prepare them until after the summer of 1943. By not developing a training program for the nurses in preparation for war, the Army projected the assumption that Army nurses were expected to staff hospitals in a civilian-like environment.

Only after nurses returned from actual battlefield conditions with descriptions of their living conditions in the war zones did the Army respond by establishing basic training camps for the nurses and designing more practical clothing for their use. Perhaps the Army wanted to perpetuate the illusion that the nurses would be safe by not training them in the art of survival. Or, perhaps planners in the War Department felt nurses would not volunteer for service if their safety was in question. Actually, training and preparation created a more competent and confident Army nurse.

By the end of the war, the Army no longer made arbitrary assignments under an air of mystery. Rather, the Army selected team members carefully to assure a proper ratio of surgical nurses, anesthetists, and medical nurses and each nurse knew whether she was assigned to a general hospital, an evacuation hospital, or a surgical field unit. Knowing more about her prospective situation produced an Army nurse who could apply more energy to her major task which was caring for the injured soldier - and less to speculation about her fate.

The nurses' exemplary efforts during the war became the basis upon which organized nursing subsequently constructed its campaign to elevate its professional status. Nurses returned home, after contributing to the Allied victory, anticipating improved, more democratic conditions in the work place. After all, the whole point of fighting the war was to guard freedom and protect democracy. Attempts by nurses to secure concessions in the postwar workplace based on these ideals, is examined in the following chapter.

Chapter Four

Homeward Bound:
Post War Plans and the
Paradox of Professionalism

B efore the Second World War ended, top nursing officials predicted a postwar nursing shortage. Unlike the factories that began to "roll up the welcome mat" for their female employees at the end of the war, the nursing profession needed to keep its members active in the work force. Employers in industry were not the only group that viewed female employees as temporary solutions to a workforce reduced when men went to war. When surveyed, the general population also believed women working in civilian jobs should return home after the war ended. This sentiment did not carry over for the nurses who were already performing traditional feminine duties. Society typically accepted nurses who worked as part of the glorification of motherhood and domesticity that continued through the postwar period. But, being content with this traditional definition of nursing prevented nurses from moving beyond a self-sacrificing role.

To retain the experienced nurses and attract new women into nursing after the war, the ANA made plans to capitalize on the position of importance nurses had occupied during the war. The ANA devised a course of action to improve the professional status of nurses in the work place and in the community. Nurses returning from the war were more confident in their skills and their abilities, and they were reluctant to return to personnel practices that exploited them. In order to attract wartime nurses to civilian positions in hospitals and clinics, nursing leaders designed policies that, when implemented, would improve civilian work place conditions and elevate each nurse's professional status.

As was true for World War I, the postwar years of World War II did indeed bring a shortage of nurses. The shortage occurred as a result of both attrition and increased demand. Civilian nurses were needed at home to care for the wounded veterans, and military nurses were needed abroad to participate in the rebuilding processes in war-torn Europe and Asia.

A demand for nurses employed in hospitals increased as hospitals became more desirable places to seek medical care. During the war years, the tendency for people to seek treatment in hospitals accelerated as a response to Social Security and the advent of affordable pre-paid group hospital plans. All of these conditions served to create more employment opportunities in nursing care, rather than reducing them as some of the returning nurses feared. Nursing leaders, therefore, directed their energies toward attaining two interdependent goals:

(1) Influence the experienced nurse to continue in civilian nursing

(2) Establish more prestige for the nursing profession

In this way, it was hoped that current active nurses could be retained and eligible young women could be appealed to join the profession. And to succeed in reaching the stated goals, the ANA purposely sought the advice of social scientists about how nursing could capitalize upon the preferred position they felt they had earned during the war. To plan better for the future of the nursing profession, and to understand more completely the intentions of the returning Army nurses, the ANA used the tools of social science that had served it well during the war. The ANA commissioned a comprehensive opinion survey to determine the postwar interests of the service nurses. This knowledge helped them plan for the future needs of nurses returning to the domestic front.

To convince the Army nurses to participate in the comprehensive survey, Katherine Densford, President of the American Nurses Association, stated in *The Journal*:

> *...your government and your fellow nurses are actively planning for the time when most of you will be returning to civilian life. Many of you are undoubtedly looking forward to home-making, but we assume that many of you are expecting to return to some type of active nursing. We need to know what you would like to do when you return. We who are trying to plan on the homefront need to know what you are thinking about and hoping for. Please use the questionnaire which will be sent you to tell us.*

The article continued to describe the nation's new appreciation of nursing:

> *It [the nation] wants more nursing service than it has ever had. It wants much more public health nursing. It wants much more of some special types of hospital service. ...we need far more well-qualified teachers than we have ever had. Your ambitions and the nation's needs are powerful incentives to more spacious planning than we have ever done. So, please fill out the questionnaire!*

The ANA sent all Army nurses the survey questionnaire. *(A table of the results of this questionnaire can be found in the Appendix.)* The typical respondent was 30 years old or younger, in the Reserves, and had served two and a half years in the Army. Sixty-nine percent of these nurses planned to remain in nursing after the war. Their replies reflected enthusiasm and optimism about the future of their careers. Of the nurses who indicated a desire to continue in nursing, 16 percent wanted to continue in the Army Nurse Corps where they felt they could advance under fairer conditions than in civilian practice. The Veterans Administration attracted 17 percent of the respondents who wanted to continue their work with injured soldiers, but 37 percent expressed interest in working as civilian nurses. Only 17 percent of all the respondents showed interest in returning to their prewar positions. Many of the active duty nurses, though, had held no employed positions before the war except perhaps that of student. Others who planned to remain active in the nursing profession sought to improve their professional status by taking advantage of educational benefits provided under the G.I. Bill of Rights. Finally, a quarter of the respondents indicated they wanted to leave the profession altogether. The remaining 6% did not answer the question. Also, it should be noted that this survey reached many nurses before hostilities had ended making it difficult for individuals to plan very far into their future.

Exhibiting excitement in anticipation of new challenges in their future, the largest group of returnees (35.5%) wanted to work in hospitals, which were becoming the major employers of nurses. Almost half of the returnees wanted additional preparation in their chosen field (46%). Although additional education would eventually improve standards of the profession, paradoxically, it would also prolong the shortage of experienced nurses actively involved in the profession. A shortage of nurses would mean inadequate service and care for patients which would in turn reflect poorly on nurses' attempts to improve their status. After nurses completed their additional education, though, patients would benefit considerably from the new graduates' advanced medical knowledge.

While nursing leaders planned the future of the profession, individual Army nurses still overseas at the end of the war, found it difficult to make long term plans. One nurse said, "We've learned in combat to live for each day and let the future take care of itself." Nurses overseas projected various reasons for choosing to leave the nursing profession after the war and some of their letters to the editor in *The Journal* reflected an attitude of resignation. For example, one nurse wrote:

> *Every nurse I have contacted over here has one desire - to go home and start her own*

family. We shall not return to the field of nursing. Many of us have given years to the profession we love. When the war ceases we'll want to have our share of peace in our own little niche. There will be a period of rehabilitation and perhaps we'll enter into that for a while - until our men get home from all over the world - but after that we'll hope to be good wives and mothers. I shall not return to nursing unless there is a dire emergency. I've learned more over here than I every dreamed I would, but I believe we have earned our right to choose our life after the war.

And, another nurse shared this optimistic opinion with *Journal* readers:

After the war, I intend to go back and start right in where I broke off. At this stage of the war, too few nurses are making any plans to return to civilian duty. Some have married, some are planning to be married at the close of the war while others merely have hopes of such. Some of them are very serious in their indifference to present-day nursing problems and trends at home. Some are seriously trying to keep pace with the nursing situation in civilian life and planning for their return to the ranks of the RN. Others are contemplating an Army career and plan to transfer to the regular army. Some are interested in the reconstruction programs to be worked out in Europe and are looking

*ahead for an opportunity to be assigned to
this service. I believe that the best days of
professional nurses are yet to be. Our
country should never suffer again for trained
nursing care. For, when this war is over,
there will be enough nurses on active duty
status to care for all.*

Nurses received intense satisfaction in caring for the men wounded in the war. As patients, soldiers injured in the war projected courage and a grateful attitude towards the nurses throughout their treatment. In contrast, nurses remembered patients at home who complained about minor discomforts. Army nurses felt they were contributing something truly worthwhile to establish world peace. They felt important, valued and essential while operating the combat zone hospitals - more so than in civilian life. Nurses also felt satisfaction in being allowed to use their "ingenuity and individuality" to solve problems and many nurses admitted it would be difficult to return to the monotony and routine of civilian nursing after experiencing the autonomy of practicing procedures typically performed by interns in civilian hospitals. Army nurses were afraid they would grow restless in civilian life and would miss the esprit de corps and "strong family spirit" that developed within their units.

The G.I. Bill of Rights assisted the nurses who wished to further their careers by earning advanced degrees, especially in public health and psychiatry. Other nurses expressed uncertainty about the future and wondered whether jobs would be available to them and other GIs when they returned home. They were apprehensive that the market would be glutted by demobilized military nurses and the new graduates of schools of nursing. In short, nurses were afraid of a repeat of the economic conditions that plagued the nursing profession during the Depression.

To counteract nurses' apprehensions about employment prospects, and in an effort to keep them in the profession after the war, the ANA publicized extensive information about the Service Extension Act of 1941 and the veterans' benefits to which nurses in the military would be entitled as civilians. The Act extended reemployment privileges of the Selective Training and Service Act of 1940 to nurses who entered active military service subsequent to May 1, 1940 which included the right to resume one's prewar job, if so desired, and if certain qualifications were met. To receive veteran's benefits, nurses had to retain their separation papers including a Certificate of Service, a Report of Separation, Separation Orders and a Letter of Appointment. These papers were the evidence of the nurses' military service that supported applications for veterans' benefits. To be eligible for education under the G.I. Bill, the applicant had to have been in the service between September 16, 1940 and the date of termination of the war.

Upon satisfying certain conditions, nurses were eligible for disability benefits, dependent allowance, medical coverage, retirement pay, pensions, Veterans Preference in the U.S. Civil Service Commission (especially the U.S. Public Health Service, Veteran Administration, and Indian Service of the Department of the Interior). Other benefits for which the nurses could qualify, included being hospitalized or receiving domiciliary care in facilities operated by the Veterans Administration. All nurses who served actively between December 7, 1941 and termination of the war, and who were discharged or retired under honorable conditions were entitled to this service. However, if the nurse's illness was not related to her service assignment, the nurse would be required to prove her inability to pay for such hospitalization. Even though veterans' benefits were the right of every nurse, the nursing leadership cautioned the veteran nurse that veterans' rights and privileges do not mean "the government is going to do all of our thinking and planning for us. The world doesn't owe us a living simply because we have donned a uniform to fight for those principles and rights which are the very backbone of our nation."

A rather large group of nurses who wanted to continue in the nursing field elected to remain in the Army Nurse Corps after the war in spite of being "variously laughed at, berated by our departing colleagues as unwilling to face the future, and told that we're making a great mistake in failing to find ourselves a place in the new fertile field of civilian nursing." But nurses found very sound reasons for continuing to serve in the ANC after the war. During the course of the war, the Army had become an organization that offered challenging opportunities to nurses, especially in the fields of reconstructive surgery and post-traumatic casualty care. In addition, it implemented personnel policies that provided job security, care during illness, leave time, retirement, travel opportunities and adventure. In the Army, general staff nurses felt as if they commanded respect by the pay, rank and status they were able to earn.

As a result of the information received from the survey, the Nursing Service of the American Red Cross predicted the profession would lose from 15,000 to 18,600 nurses during the transition from military to civilian status. To deal with the shortage, the ANA urged teaching institutions to prepare for the estimated 40,000 nurses who were returning for advanced educational preparation. The ANA also wanted to take a regional approach to planning and distribution and therefore urged state associations to determine the number of nurses they could anticipate returning to a nursing position in their area. Realizing that a nurse shortage would damage the positive image they received during the war, nursing advocates prompted nurses to become actively involved in the health insurance movement in order to assure the profession and its members a higher level of usefulness, and economic security.

Nursing leaders used the public relations contacts they made during the war and sought their expert advice on a course of action and direction for organized nursing. Edward Bernays, a well-known publicist, represented the public relations firm that advised the ANA. He explained that to increase its prestige and status, the nursing profession had to meet the real needs of the public for nursing services. According to Bernays, three distinct publics interacted with nursing: the government public, the medical public, and the patient public; and relations must be good with all three. To meet the needs of these constituents, a public relations strategy would educate the public about nursing and direct nursing to meet the legitimate needs of the public. That is, organized nursing needed to be guided by and lead public opinion - simultaneously.

To improve the public's understanding of the nursing profession, Bernays attempted to find out the difference between what the public expected of nursing and what the public believed it was getting. Bernays determined how the "public" thought by surveying, what he called, public opinion molders such as newspaper and magazine editors, radio commentators, news photographers, cartoonists, columnists, authors, radio script writers, book publishers, lecturers, artists, and illustrators. Bernays argued that these groups' opinions about nursing would "largely reflect [nursing's] standing with the public... As these men and women speak and write, so the public mind is affected."

Bernays found conflicting sentiments about nursing among the opinion molders. Results of his survey showed that the respondents had a "very high regard" for the women performing nursing services, especially their contribution to the war effort, but believed the cost of nursing was too high. Criticisms for the profession related to the public's perception of nurses' education, and individual encounters with nurses who they felt were lazy and lacked human sympathy, believing there was room for improvement in their interpersonal skills. Finally, the opinion molders emphasized the need of a public relations program, greater psychological understanding of patients by the nurses, and economic adjustments for the profession.

In order to bring about these changes, the public opinion shapers made some thoughtful suggestions. First of all, organized nursing should either hire a good public relations firm or set up an in-house public relations department. Then it should disseminate information regarding the training of nurses including the cost and time of preparation for licensing by publishing more articles in popular magazines like *Life*. According to Bernays, nursing leaders would find it helpful to make available more facts about the differences between practical and registered nurses to the public and publicize more praise from the doctors.

In all the public relations material, the emphasis should be on nurses as professionals, not as diagnosticians or as servants. And finally, Bernays suggested that efforts should be made to "recruit finer women into the profession," a statement which is unclear in its meaning to the author. Bernays also instructed the profession to "sustain, intensify, and utilize" the huge reservoir of good will war veterans felt toward them by participating in veteran-related activities and taking on leadership roles in the Veterans Administration. In following this advice,

Bernays declared, the nursing profession could advance its own interests while performing a valuable public service.

―――――――――――――――――

While official nursing groups worked to capitalize on the war service rendered by individual nurses, individual nurses who returned from the combat zone contemplated the importance and effectiveness of their participation in and contributions to the war effort and attempted to effect positive changes for their individual circumstances at work. One nurse claimed that "a great deal of good for nursing came out of the war." Army and Navy nurses had become well prepared in surgery, psychiatry, orthopedics, physiotherapy, and other areas of medical science. With this knowledge, and the short cuts and speed Army nurses acquired under combat conditions, they could certainly apply these life-saving skills successfully in civilian hospitals. The ex-service nurses who wanted to stay in nursing generally felt that they would return from the war stronger both physically and mentally and would approach their postwar days as more calm and composed individuals because of the ordeals they had faced overseas.

As a result of the self-esteem and confidence in their abilities nurses developed during their wartime experiences, they gave serious consideration to the working conditions to which they would return after the war. One nurse admitted that before serving in the Army Nurse Corps she and her friends did not recognize inequitable personnel practices. But after time and distance away from their previous work situations, these same nurses realized that "certain personnel practices become glaringly wrong and unfair." Nurses wanted higher professional standards, adequate salaries to provide for an appropriate standard of living, job security, and time to participate in outside activities.

Not all nurses concerned themselves with the material compensations of work. One nurse wrote about the intrinsic rewards of nursing as a self-sacrificing calling, saying that four things keep nurses in nursing:

1. Pride

2. A sense of moral obligation to the profession

3. Inertia

4. The fact that bedside care is "one of the most natural, satisfying experiences to which a woman can devote herself."

Regardless of outlook, returning nurses and nurses who remained on the homefront would once again be working together and both groups knew they would have to resolve workplace conflicts. In anticipation of conflicts that might occur between the two groups, *The Journal* carried a variety of articles and personal testimonies that addressed the situation. One article in particular offered advice for defusing potential friction. In it, the author suggested that returning nurses should express openly to their co-workers their changed attitudes, points of view, and altered expectations that developed as a result of wartime experiences. Homeward bound nurses hoped civilian nurses would "greet them with understanding, sympathy, and the spirit of helpfulness to get them back to a normal life."

Ex-service nurses believed they shared common outlooks among themselves after sharing common experiences. They had eaten the same institutional food, and would therefore "like ice-cream and green salads in the same proportion that they disliked spam and dehydrated potatoes." They had also shared camp life, homesickness, and the broadening effect of international travel.

Nurses who had worked in field hospitals and evacuation units felt they had changed the most. One observer described the typical experience of field nurses:

> ...they have nearly all worked under enemy fire, have lived under field conditions, and have been constantly on the move; these nurses had fewer rules and regulations than the usual nurses. They developed, therefore, a sense of independence and initiative which is not typical of the traditional nurse. All this makes this group more weary, more restless, and will make their readjustment more difficult.

Experiences of nurses who worked in general hospitals overseas, however, resembled more closely civilian nurses' practices on the homefront and therefore required less transition time than the field nurse.

Regardless of their wartime service, however, veteran nurses wanted rest and time to recuperate more than anything else before returning to active civilian duty. By the time she returned to the states, she would have recovered from the immediate effects of battle fatigue but the longer-lasting effects of "nervousness" accumulated from "life in a fox-hole and under shell fire" took longer to conquer. Some returning nurses believed that their experiences resulted in personality changes making them at once "more self-assured, more fatalistic, and sometimes more smug" as a result of being involved firsthand with the gruesome realities of war. Upon their return, ex-service nurses requested time to do some indulgent living. These indulgences were really very commonplace and included sleeping in a silk nightgown once again, using an indoor bathroom with plumbing, and enjoying an ice cream soda with friends.

In all fairness, it must be stated that ex-service nurses were not always aware of, or sensitive to the harsh and austere conditions under which homefront nurses worked. At times they failed to understand the difficulties civilian nurses endured during the war and their contributions toward winning the war. Civilian nurses had carried a heavy burden at home and expected some relief when the war ended. Without this consideration, cooperation in the workplace between returning military nurses and civilian nurses became difficult and at times little recognition for each group's point of view existed.

Battlefield conditions produced nurses with "a sense of independence and initiative which is not typical of the traditional nurse," declared one nurse. Nurses could have incorporated their new-found qualities of independence and initiative into their patient care philosophy instead of interpreting their growth as an impediment to readjustment in civilian life and in medicine. Civilian nurses felt military nurses failed to appreciate their efforts and sacrifices made on the homefront and military nurses felt medical care in civilian hospitals focused on alleviating petty ailments. Altogether, a workplace environment with these misunderstandings created an atmosphere of resentment in some work places.

Ex-military service nurses who were returning to civilian positions expected more job satisfaction and more financial remuneration for their work than they had expected before the war. Nurses who had served overseas and risked their lives felt that they had the right to be more selective and discriminating in choosing their future life course instead of leaving important decisions to others. They had been "fighting for democracy and found that our profession was far behind in enjoying the recognition as well as the rights and privileges of a democracy..."

Civilian nurses and nurses re-entering the civilian work place after military service, therefore, shared complaints concerning inadequate salary, paltry health care programs, inadequate vacation and sick leave policies and few opportunities to advance. Additionally, the absence of clearly written or well-defined employment policies caused confusion and frustration in an environment where the employees believed the work was too hard, patients were too demanding, work schedules were too long and not planned far enough ahead, and did not include shared or rotated shift-work. Finally, the nurses perceived the administration as autocratic, narrow-minded, and biased.

When comparing themselves with other female-dominated occupations, nurses often found that women in these other fields required less education, worked fewer days, earned higher salaries, were eligible for more vacation days, and had fewer responsibilities. Many nurses held the opinion that until their profession was treated with higher respect, commanded a higher salary and enjoyed better working conditions, nurses would continue to be indifferent to the nurse shortage.

Nurses also discovered that the Registered Nurse designation was "professional" in name only since they were not consistently treated so by the physicians with whom they worked. One nurse commented:

> *I feel a little more understanding and a little more kindness and consideration from doctors and hospital executives would have prevented the present shortage of nurses.*

Another nurse expressed frustration at being criticized for "the small things" by physicians rather than being recognized and encouraged for "the daily load carried by each nurse that is so heavy... ." Many nurses were made to feel as if they were "doing nothing."

Upon their return from a successful wartime career, ex-service nurses found that they had to return once again to an environment in which blind obedience to the physician and uncomplaining acceptance of criticism were routine. They felt as if they had returned to student-like status rather than the professional status they anticipated. Veteran nurses expected to return to an environment that encouraged a spirit of cooperative effort, (not unlike the team effort they enjoyed during the war) and participation in the planning and decision-making process that affected their careers.

The ANA reacted to this general attitude by developing and adopting ten resolutions in September 1946 that established a guide for improving and elevating the status of the nursing profession and each member therein. The ANA resolved to:

1. Improve hours and living conditions; including a 40-hour work week with no decrease in salary, a "minimum wage net" to attract quality nurses and to provide a certain standard of living comparable with other professions.

2. Provide and improve community health programs.

3. Increase participation by nurses in planning and administration of nursing services in hospitals.

4. Use professional associations for collective bargaining and negotiations affecting employment practices.

5. Remove employment and development barriers against racial minorities.

6. Implement state licensing of PNs and auxiliary workers.

7. Improve counseling and placement services for nurses creating greater job stability and satisfaction.

8. Develop pre-pay health and medical care plans to include nursing care.

9. Maintain educational standards through continuing education subsidized by federal and foundation funds.

10. Conduct self-appraisals by national nursing organizations and act upon such appraisals to improve the profession.

As nursing leaders worked toward professionalization, salary became a central issue. The American Nurses' Association studied the salaries of 226,520 general staff nurses in the fall of 1942. At that time the median annual salary, in addition to full maintenance, was $981 (which included provisions for room and board). If partial maintenance was provided, the median salary was $1,141. A staff nurse earned a median salary of $1,200 if no maintenance was paid. In contrast, nurses in the military who volunteered for foreign service earned $108 per month or about $1296 per year in salary - twenty percent higher than nurses staying on the homefront. That is to say, military nurses serving stateside would earn an average of $18 per month less than nurses overseas.

After the war, nurses compared their salaries with other traditional female occupations. One nurse complained that returning to her prewar nursing position would pay $110 a month (about $100 take-home) while a department store offered $160 a month, telephone operators made $154 a month and typists and stenographers could earn from $130 to $195 a month. In other words, nurses earned approximately 74 cents an hour compared with 97 cents an hour for typists, $1.11 per hour for bookkeepers and $1.32 per hour for seamstresses.

Additionally, women in these positions typically worked a 40- or 44-hour week in contrast to the 48-hour week nurses worked, and they enjoyed opportunities for regular salary increases, promotions, and health and pension benefits to which nurses usually did not have access.

Individual nurses were aware of their salary inequities and wanted the disparities to be addressed. Yet spokeswomen for the nursing profession communicated conflicting attitudes on wage compensations. Although they were trying to elevate their status by suggesting a "minimum wage net" as part of their Resolutions, nursing leaders continued to maintain a service outlook that undermined a militant stance on the issue of wages. However, this attitude was contrary to the advice that the public relations experts and some physician-advocates gave them: "since nurses must live by their labor, they cannot give their services gratuitously." But the ANA wanted to develop the concept of nursing as a "self-motivating profession capable of growth and adjustment rather than a mere service to be sold in the market place." The editor of the *American Journal of Nursing*, Mary Roberts, scolded the nurses who were concerned about wages and who appeared to be more interested in "selling their services to the highest bidder than about making the best use of their professional skill less they sell their birthright for a mess of pottage *[sic]*." Policy-makers in nursing organizations firmly maintained that to dwell on salary was "contrary to the fundamental American concept of the nurse" and believed emphasizing salary increases would have a disastrous influence on the profession.

Another issue related to improving the prestige of nursing concerned education, and once again illustrates the confusing messages nursing leaders issued. The National League of Nursing Education began working in 1943 to develop advanced courses in clinical nursing. The NLNE focused especially on courses that veteran nurses could take under the G.I. Bill. By taking these courses, nurses "could do much to promote the prestige and to improve the standards of bedside nursing. In this way they would help to provide valid arguments for better financial rewards."

In order to attract more women to nursing, the Higher Education and National Defense Committee of the American Council on Education advised and directed women to adopt "feminine" occupations like nursing and other "welfare" fields rather than physics and mathematics since "it is women educated in these [feminine] fields who will probably be the most useful in postwar reconstruction work at home and abroad." *(Other 'welfare' occupations included those in public health, nutrition, and recreation.)* In fact, considerable press was dedicated to projecting the message that women in "men's jobs" should relinquish them as the warriors returned home. The need for workers in low-paying non-skilled positions and in traditionally female occupations, however, continued to grow in the postwar economy.

Nursing leaders recognized the climate of demand for women's participation in the work force as another opportunity to elevate their status. Once again they invited the public relations expert, Edward Bernays, to consider and advise them on the issue of whether nurses could be considered full-fledged professionals. Bernays asked a group of social scientists to define the elements that constitute a "profession" and determine if nurses could be included within that definition. Nursing's propensity to occupy an ambiguous position in the world of work and within medicine succeeded in evoking diametrically opposing views by the experts. Social scientists could not agree upon whether or not nursing could be considered a profession. Those who identified nursing as a profession stated that nurses possessed elements necessary for professional status such as "a fundamental body of scientific knowledge, thorough educational training, and the licensure by the state without which a nurse cannot practice." But those who placed nursing outside the professional arena stated that the public perceived nurses as "menial workers who are completely subordinated to doctors, and do not command high enough pay to maintain professional status."

Bernays concluded that:

> *...technically the nurse is professional, but she cannot achieve true professional status until she raises her prestige. Prestige results from demonstrable competence in nursing, higher salaries, evidence of greater interest in public affairs, and more independence.*

Prestige could not be won, however, as long as the postwar nursing shortage continued, patients perceived that they received inadequate nursing care, and physicians refused to recognize nurses and nurses' duties and responsibilities as equal to their own duties and functions.

Organized nursing failed to win approval from physicians for their aspirations to become professionals. Nursing leaders could have used the nurse shortage as a catalyst for change in standards for established registered nurses by using the developing category of auxiliary workers, especially practical nurses (PNs), to elevate them into a status nearer that of physicians. In bringing this new classification of health care worker under their direction, registered nurses could have distinguished themselves from a group of nonprofessionals and diverted the more menial and unpleasant duties away from their scope of responsibility.

Nursing leaders were unable to exploit the conditions under which auxiliary personnel became more established because physicians used auxiliaries to place nurses on the defensive. In fact, the presence of the auxiliary workers created a debate around the possibility of RNs educating themselves out of a job. This was the opinion of Dr. Frank Lahey, former president of the American Medical Association as well as many hospital administrators.

Many physicians exhibited little respect for nursing in general, especially in their published writings concerning nurses' position and status in medicine. Physicians felt nursing duties could be performed by auxiliary workers with little formal training. In a survey made by the American College of Surgeons, 84% of the responding surgeons indicated that nursing care could be provided by "auxiliary help" rather than a professionally educated nursing staff. Whereas the growth of practical nurses actually began as an expedient response to the wartime shortage of nurses at home, the trend continued to develop during the postwar shortage as well. The trend created a backlash against the professionalizing efforts of organized nursing. One hospital administrator wrote:

> *Nurses should either get off their high horses and do the physical work they started out to do or move over and let others do it. There is too much talk about high professional standards' and not enough about taking care of the sick.*

The president of the American Medical Association held a similar view. In his opinion, nurses were "legislating and educating themselves out of jobs." Another prominent physician predicted that nurses with degrees would lose their jobs to practical nurses because "one definitely does not need a Ph.D. degree to carry a bedpan. The patients are only interested in whether it is hot or cold."

These physicians were unwilling to acknowledge the important functions performed by an educated force of nurses. Their shortsightedness in realizing the usefulness of associates, the caliber to which nurses aspired by adhering to strict standards of education, arose from their fear of having to contend with a competing group of health care professionals. Physicians wanted a force of passive recipients for their orders and prescriptions. Nurses, however, spent more time with individual patients, and with their broad medical background, were capable of making a knowledgeable contribution on behalf of the patient's needs.

Physicians perceived nurses' aspirations as conflicting with their sphere of authority. Rather than accepting the situation as one of cooperation that would benefit the patient, physicians held on to their monopoly in medicine by withholding approval of nurses as professionals. This judgment cost patients the potential for innovative care strategies on their behalf. Unable to confront their doubts and uncertainties about their own status, physicians protected their preserve by publicly detracting from nurses' merits and pitted them against auxiliary workers by generating employment insecurities. Physicians possessed more power than nurses and controlled the use of auxiliary personnel. In fact, physicians used the auxiliary personnel as a weapon to prevent registered nurses from expanding their authority.

The ANA, along with many of the rank-and-file nurses, disagreed with physicians' opinions about them, especially concerning their own education. In fact, during the war and after, a noticeable trend developed in nursing schools. The number of schools of nursing associated with a college or university increased. That increase was accompanied by a growth in enrollment in programs that led to a bachelor's degree in nursing rather than a diploma or certificate.

Between the end of World War II and the Korean Conflict, the nursing profession worked to effect positive changes for its members. The ANA continued to debate the issue of professionalization and the related issues of salary and education until 1950 when the Korean Conflict suddenly diverted its attention. Nursing leaders did not have the time to prepare for reserve recruitment as they did prior to World War II. They anticipated another major war and confronted the possibilities of a nuclear attack on American soil. Nursing leaders predicted that a "mass exodus" of civilian nurses to the military would have "dire consequences" on health care at home.

During this time, however, while civilian nursing struggled for any advancements they realized, the military's nursing corps progressed fairly smoothly in upgrading its personnel practices. Ironically, nursing leaders had successfully compelled the military to remove many of the restrictions that inhibited nurses' efforts early in the war. For example, Congress awarded commissioned grades to members of the Army and Navy Nurse Corps in 1947. By the time the Army Nurse Corps began expanding for duty in Korea, it was using male nurses, minorities and auxiliary workers to lessen demands on the RNs. Because of the changes in clothing, training and assignments that took place during World War II, nurses who served in Korea entered active duty areas better prepared for wartime nursing than at the beginning of World War II. Nursing care for the Korean conflict was directed by the Joint Committee on Nursing in National Security, a more efficient and productive organization than the committees that functioned during World War II.

After 1947, responsibility for recruiting and maintaining a reserve of nurses fell to the Army rather than the American Red Cross Nursing Service as in past wars. The Army organized, matched and distributed nurses with various backgrounds to appropriate medical units in the Army Nurse Corps so that specific skills were utilized to the best advantage. Members of the ANC commanded the respect accorded all officers, and administrators adopted enlightened personnel policies that allowed for generous vacation and sick leave, medical attention, and retirement benefits.

These were the very concessions civilian nursing leaders had been striving to obtain for themselves. And even though the medical profession used nurses to meet the increased demands in healthcare by allowing them to actively participate in the use of diagnostics, antibiotics or "miracle drugs", and other post war medical advancements in thoracic, orthopedic, and internal medicine, personnel policies failed to keep pace with and reward the nurses' improvements in expertise. The average work week was reduced by only two hours in five years, from 48 hours in 1941 to 46 hours in 1946. And although nurses realized a slight increase in salaries after the war, they were not comparable to other professions.

Nursing leaders, therefore, realized only part of their vision they held for the profession. In the areas where nursing leaders had control, especially in education, they were able to make considerable progress. But outside that sphere, such as in hospital administration and personnel administration where they were not in control, nurses realized little progress in policy changes, and they met with reluctance to any changes at all, in some cases. The medical profession felt threatened and intimidated by the nurses' demands and as the group in power, they were unwilling to relinquish any of it to a group they viewed as inferior.

World War II provided an opportunity for nurses to prove their critical importance but nursing leaders found it difficult to maintain their gains in time of peace when their skills were once again a mere commodity to be exploited in the free market. Nursing encountered insurmountable barriers to professionalization from various directions. Physicians, as males and as the dominant health-brokers, were threatened by competition from the nurses. They wielded considerable power through the AMA and prevented any inroads into their territory.

The very nature of nursing itself lent itself to classification among the semi-professions. Many nurses liked the feminine nature of their profession but as a result, the field remained as subordinate to medicine as women were to men. Nurses lacked the power to demand concessions within the medical hierarchy. Nevertheless, organized nursing was led by a group of intelligent and talented women who recognized the importance of their contribution to the war effort. The potential to transfer their considerable skills to benefit the general public could have gained more power for organized nursing in terms of bargaining for higher status, if not the prestige of a full-fledged professional. They failed because they placed too much importance on the "nobleness" of their vocation, a vague and nebulous quality, and therefore difficult to reward. If recognizing nursing as a "calling" maintained such importance for nursing, perhaps those working for advancement would have succeeded if they had sought to articulate why *caring* was just as important in health care as *curing*. At this critical crossroad, perhaps nursing leaders should have worked to convince physicians, hospital administrators, public relations experts and the general public that the art of caring, exercised with scientific theory and practice deserved greater prestige and compensations.

Chapter Five

Conclusions

Florence Nightingale emerged as the dominant character in nursing folklore during the Crimean War. Nightingale embodied the image of nursing as a genteel calling of womanly devotion to healing through service and nurture. Since her appearance, each successive generation of nurses has worked to increase organized nursing's prominence within the world of medicine. Following the Victorian traditions of Nightingale and other pioneers in nineteenth-century nursing, a group of elite nursing leaders during World War II directed an entire population of active nurses to cover the healthcare needs of civilians at home and the fighting men at war.

Nursing leaders in World War II came from the ranks of nurses who had participated in the First World War and they used their experiences to pursue higher status and prestige for nursing by capitalizing on nurses' contributions to the war efforts. Although nursing leaders relied heavily on the Victorian definition of nursing, they were sophisticated enough to know that since nursing was a strategic defense skill and essential for military victory, war could be used to elevate their status. War emergencies created opportunities for advancement in technology and medicine. Educators in nursing schools kept current with these developments in medicine and employed them in their curricula. Codes of behavior remained strict, however, and emphasis on gender-based role expectations for nurses never changed.

Organized nursing encountered, and yet surmounted the barriers and restrictions thrust upon them by government and military officials. Nursing organizations competed with civilian industries for recruits. Early in the war, recruiters relied upon one-to-one contact, posters, pamphlets, exhibits and displays at the community level. Later, nurse recruiters gained access to the skills of the federally backed advertising industry to broadcast the message that more nurses needed to volunteer for active service at home and abroad. Popular media and professional journals transferred the responsibility for soldiers' safety and well-being on to women in the factories and in nursing, claiming that men would die needlessly without their dedicated work. Propaganda stressed the intrinsic and traditional rewards of nursing rather than its professional and technical nature.

The all-volunteer basis of recruiting for the nursing corps limited recruitment efforts as did marriage and age restrictions. With the support of the rank-and-file nurses, nursing leaders eventually convinced the Army to lift those barriers and open military opportunities to more women. Removing the marriage and age barrier constraints facilitated filling quotas for active military nurses issued by the Army. Meeting the Army's quota demands was no small feat for the nursing leaders who worked with a smaller recruitment budget than other agencies, such as the Women's Army Corps.

Initially, the Army did not adequately prepare the nurse recruit for operating under wartime conditions or issue her the essential gear for doing her job. The nursing leadership, again, succeeded in establishing a training program for each nurse to attend before she embarked upon her adventure. By the end of the war, nurses going into the Army underwent a course of training that prepared them for combat conditions and created enthusiasm within the nurse corps for their mission. And although the field nurses who went to war without benefit of this training relied on their own initiative in enduring hardships and scavenging for necessities, preparation made a difference. Boot camp training produced nurses who were more confident in their abilities. Issuing proper gear to nurses allowed them to direct more energy toward skill utilization and less into the day-to-day drudgery of survival.

Being placed in units for which they were specifically trained meant nurses' skills were employed more efficiently. And being briefed about their particular type of duty assignment meant nurses could prepare mentally for their destination. Expecting Army nurses to work under mysterious conditions was a patronizing manner for the Army to treat professional military officers.

As the Army Nurse Corps followed each combat unit to the battlefront, nurses filled many roles in addition to that of healer. Some military strategists even felt that nurses' nurturing and morale-building function was strategic to victory and used that as an excuse to justify placing nurses in mortal danger. Nurses who served overseas were overextended in treating the wounded, but they enjoyed the latitude to improvise, experiment and take responsibility for tasks they would not have been able to perform during peace time.

Individual nurses returned from the war confident in themselves and in their abilities, and ready to demand respect, status, prestige, higher wages, better benefits, and improved work place conditions. Recognition of their own abilities created an element of rising expectations for the nurses' future. For those nurses who served in the war, their experiences made them see how unfairly they had been treated in the work place relative to the importance of their skills to society's healthcare needs. Although essential during both war and peace, nurses' contributions were undervalued by physicians, hospital administrators, and patients at home. Upon their return to civilian nursing, nurses expected no less than better work conditions in which they could use the skills and abilities they acquired in the war.

After the war ended and factory owners began dismissing women from their wartime jobs, nursing leaders encouraged nurses to remain employed as nurses. Some nurses left their careers behind them upon returning home. Most nurses, though, were enthusiastic about opportunities to further their careers through higher education and through advanced training programs offered as part of the G.I. Bill of Rights. Nurses who remained in nursing after the war found that work place conflicts developed between the nurses who served at home and those who served overseas. Through a spirit of cooperation and understanding, however, nurses in both groups were able to resolve much of the friction.

Returning nurses wanted more democratic working conditions and more equitable compensations after sacrificing their time and talents for their country. These same nurses were now unwilling to allow their employers to exploit them as in the past. Nursing leaders addressed these demands through various professional associations, most notably, the American Nurses Association. Officials in the ANA consulted social scientists and advocate doctors for advice about the future of nursing. Nursing leaders chose to remain true to the traditions upon which nursing was founded. This choice prevented them from blazing new directions until after the Victorian ideologies upon which nursing policies were based were no longer an overwhelming influence.

A new category of nurse developed during the war - the auxiliary or practical nurse. Nurses and physicians struggled to control this new resource. Organized nursing should have been able to use this class of health care assistants to elevate their status at least partially. In fact, auxiliary nurses and their tasks came under the jurisdiction of the nursing hierarchy, but physicians possessed the power to use auxiliary nurses as bargaining chips. That is, in order to restrain registered nurses' advancements and keep them dependent on physicians and hospital administrators for their career opportunities, doctors threatened to replace the formally educated nurse with the practical nurse. Therefore, the physicians' resistance to nurses' aspirations and the conventional attitudes of nurses worked together to inhibit substantial improvements in the nursing field.

Improvements in status also failed to keep pace with nurses' advances in experiential skills and education gained in the war because nursing is a female-dominated occupation and an occupation whose practitioners are ancillary to physicians. Nursing leaders chose to maintain a narrow definition of nursing that stressed the importance of femininity and womanhood. They also emphasized the nature of nursing as a calling - a vocation whose compensations were intrinsic rather than material. Finally, in addition to failing to secure the support and blessing of the physicians under whom they worked, nursing leaders failed to create a clearly defined mission for themselves. They emphasized education and professionalism, on one hand, but placed importance on the nurturing aspect of nursing, on the other. Organized nursing preached the gospel of professionalism while they practiced the non-professional nature of nursing: selflessness, altruism, heroism and internal satisfaction.

Young nurses who volunteered for active military service fulfilled traditional role expectations while they experienced adventure, gratitude and glory. Without having to expend extra energy competing with men, nurses were free to feel and enjoy the inner satisfaction of contributing something important to the war effort. In return, they expected a postwar future with opportunities for advancements in rank, education, and in the profession.

Nurses' failure to professionalize during World War II illustrates how gender conventions within an occupation can impede women's efforts to improve their lot. Although necessary for victory, their service was hindered by conflicts and tensions between the predominately female nursing profession and the male domain of military, government, and medical professionals. Expecting to capitalize on their contributions to the war effort after the war, organized nursing instead came head-to-head with the male medical doctors and hospital administrators opposed to elevating nurses' status.

Paradoxically, strict and disciplined nursing training, which was adapted from the nineteenth century model, facilitated nurses' endurance and accomplishments during the war. But that same Nightingale influence prevented the nursing sisterhood from attaining the goal to fully professionalize its occupation. Qualities that insured the nurses' success in the war emphasized a humanitarian approach to caring and, unfortunately, did not command the respect and rewards of a full-fledged profession. Although nursing leaders surmounted the obstacles thrown in their way during the course of the war, they were unable to overcome gender restraints inherent in their field in order to carve out a higher place for themselves in the medical hierarchy.

APPENDIX

Chart 1. The Place of Nursing in the Federal Government's Council of National Defense

The President of the United States
↓
↓

Council of National Defense
Henry L. Stimson, Secretary of War
Frank Knox, Secretary of the Navy
Harold Ickes, Secretary of the Interior
↓
↓

Coordinator of Health and Welfare
Federal Security Agency
Paul V. McNutt, Administrator
↓
↓

Health and Medical Committee
Irvin Abell, MD, Chairman
Maj. Gen. James Magee, Surgeon General, U.S. Army
Thomas Parran, MD, Surgeon General, US Public Health
Service
↓
↓

Subcommittee on Nursing
Mary Beard, RN, Chairman
Julia C. Stimson, RN
Marion Howell, RN
Nellie X. Hawkinson, RN
Sister M. Olivia Gowan, RN

Chart 2. The Organization of the Nursing Council on National Defense

Affiliated Organizations

American Nurses' Association
National League of Nursing Education
National Organization for Public Health Nursing
National Association of Colored Graduate Nurses
Association of Collegiate Schools of Nursing
American Red Cross Nursing Service

Ex Officio Members

Federal Nursing Services
Army Nurse Corps
Navy Nurse Corps
U.S. Public Health Service
U.S. Veterans Administration
Editorial Staff of the *American Journal of Nursing*
Editorial Staff of *Public Health Nursing*

Executive Committee

Julia C. Stimson, RN
Susan C. Francis, RN
Sister M. Olivia Gowan, RN
Stella Goostray, RN
Marion W. Sheahan, RN

Executive Secretary

Elmira B. Wickenden, RN

Table 1. Student Nurse Enrollment
Number Enrolled in State Accredited Schools of
Nursing
1941 – 1945

Year	Number of of Students	Number of Schools
1941	87,588	1,303
1942	91,457	1,299
1943	100,486	1,297
1944	112,249	1,307
1945	126,576	1,295

Table 2. Gallup Poll: Public Opinion Survey for February 1945

A. Do you approve/disapprove of the proposal now before Congress to draft nurses to serve with the Army and Navy?

Approve	73 %
Disapprove	19 %
No Opinion	8 %
Total	100 %

B. Do you think there is a shortage of nurses in the armed forces now?

Yes	78 %
No	2 %
No Opinion	20 %
Total	100 %

Table 3. American Red Cross Nursing Service Record of Recruitment for Army Nurse Corps during World War II

Recruitment Periods	Volunteered/ Certified	Assigned to A.N.C.	Percent Assigned
12/7/41 - 6/30/42	14,075	7,123	50.6
7/1/42 - 6/30/43	36,442	24,052	66.0
7/1/43 - 6/30/44	21,639	17,025	78.7
7/1/44 - 6/30/45	31,713	22,266	70.2
Total	103,869	70,466	67.8

Table 4. Salary of the Army Nurse Corps in 1943

Grades	Annual Base Pay	Subsistence Allowance	Rental Allowance
Colonel	$ 4,000	$ 21	$ 105
Lt. Colonel	3,500	21	105
Major	3,000	21	90
Captain	2,400	21	75
First Lt.	2,000	21	60
Second Lt.	1,800	21	45

Table 5. Age of Army Nurse Corps Nurses Responding to an ANA-Sponsored Survey May 1946

Age	Number	Percent
Under 30	18,879	60.9
30 - 39	9,610	31.0
40 and over	2,418	7.8
No Answer	93	0.3
Total	31,000	100.0

(Median age = 28.5 years)

Table 6. Status of Nurses in the Army Nurse Corps May 1946

Status	Number	Percent
Regular Army	806	2.6
Army Reserves	30,194	97.4
Total	31,000	100.0

Table 7. Length of Military Service
May 1946

Length of time	Number	Percent
One year or less	3,999	12.9
1 - 2 years	8,060	26.0
2 - 3 years	12,245	39.5
3 - 4 years	4,371	14.1
4 or more years	2,139	6.9
No Answer	186	0.6
Total	31,000	100.0

(Median length of service = 2.3 years)

Table 8. Year of Graduation from School of Nursing

Year	Number	Percent
1925 or before	1,209	3.9
1926 - 1930	2,883	9.3
1931 - 1035	4,774	15.4
1936 - 1940	8,463	27.3
1941 - 1945	12,896	41.6
No Answer	775	2.5
Total	31,000	100.0

(Median time since graduation = 6.5 years)

Table 9. Postwar Expectations in Returning to Civilian Status

Expectation	Prewar Position		Prewar State of Reg'n	
	Number	Percent	Number	Percent
Expect to return	4,960	16.0	20,460	66.0
Don't expect to return	22,630	73.0	7,037	22.7
No Answer	3,410	11.0	3,503	11.3
Total	31,000	100.0	31,000	100.0

Table 10. Field of Interest for Service and Further Preparation

Field	Service		Preparation	
	Number	Percent	Number	Percent
Public Health	4,030	13.0	3,472	11.2
Hospital	11,005	35.5	5,952	19.2
Teaching	1,240	4.0	1,085	3.5
Industrial	3,968	12.8	2,325	7.5
Private Duty	1,550	5.0	186	0.6
Foreign Service	124	0.4	93	0.3
Non-Spec'd	1,953	6.3	1,240	4.0
No Additional Preperation	-	-	16,647	53.7
No Answer	7,130	23.0	-	-
Total	31,000	100.0	31,000	100.0

203

Table 11. Number of Active Nurses

Year	Number
1930	214,189
1940	450,000
1945	526,933
1948	280,500
1949	300,533

Table 12. Nurses Employed by Hospitals

Year	Number
1930	77,000
1940	63,536*
1946	144,724
1948	167,400
1949	199,295

* ANA members only

Table 13. Nurses Employed by Federal Government

Year	Number
1930	4,703
1939	6,107
1940	7,772
1941	12,863
1944	55,337
1945	72,978
1947	21,592
1948	21,965
1949	23,791
1950	22,387

Table 14. All Nursing Schools Meeting Minimum Requirements

Year	Number
1939	1,328
1940	1,311
1944	1,307
1945	1,295
1946	1,280
1947	1,253
1948	1,245
1949	1,215
1950	1,190

Table 15. Nursing Schools Connected with Colleges or Universities

Year	Number
1939	80
1940	76
1943	120
1944	137
1945	138
1946	171
1948	183
1950	195

Table 16. Students Enrolled in Nursing Programs

Year	Number
1939	82,095
1940	85,000
1944	112,249
1945	126,576
1946	128,828
1947	106,900
1948	91,643
1949	88,817
1950	97,903

Table 17. Students Graduated from Nursing Programs

Year	Number
1938	20,655
1940	23,600
1944	28,276
1945	33,700
1946	36,195
1947	40,744
1949	21,379

Table 18. Government Supported Hospitals

Year	Number
1938	1,728
1940	1,767
1943	2,284
1944	2,262
1946	2,183
1948	372
1949	361

Table 19. Non-Government Supported Hospitals

Year	Number
1938	4,438
1940	4,524
1943	4,371
1944	4,349
1946	4,328
1948	5,963
1949	6,211

Table 20. Enrollees in Group Hospital Plans

Year	Number	
1935	75,000	
1937	600,000	
1939	2,900,000	
1941	6,149,222	
1944	4,975,850	
1946	21,359,000	*(Blue Cross only)*
	4,975,850	*(Other plans)*
1947	25,876,424	*(Blue Cross only)*
1948	29,498,527	*(Blue Cross only)*

Table 21. Typical Work Week for Staff Nurses

Year	Hours
1936	48
1941	48
1946	48
1949	40

Table 22. Annual Salaries for Staff Nurses

Year	Amount	
1934	$ 984	(median)*
1935	$ 999	(median)*
1936	$ 1,325	(median)**
1945	$ 1,800 - 2,496	(range)
1946	$ 1,000 - 2,640	(range)
	$ 1,860	(mean)
1949	$ 2,532	(mean)*

*(excludes maintenance allowance for as much
    as $500 per year)*

**(includes maintenance allowance)*

Table 23. Comparisons of Nurses' Salaries with Those of Other Business and Professional Women 1936

Occupation	Number Reporting	Median Salary	Range of Middle Half
Othr Professionals	4,692	$ 1,410	$ 1,060 - 1,880
Teachers	3,210	1,375	1,025 - 1,845
Nurses	556	1,640	1,235 - 1,980
Librarians	268	1,485	1,075 - 1,945
Office mgrs	281	1,470	1,115 - 1,970
Secretaries/ stenographers	2,604	1,270	920 - 1,665

Table 24. Number of Nurses Compared to Other Professions 1940

Professional Occupation	Number of Women	Number of Men	Total Number	Percent Women
Nurses	362,897	8,169	371,066	97.8
Lawyers/ judges	4,447	176,036	180,483	2.5
Physicians/ surgeons	7,708	157,921	165,629	4.7
Teachers	806,860	269,141	1,076,001	75.0
Social welfare/ Religious	74,423	35,946	110,369	67.4

Table 25 Military Awards as of June 30, 1945

Army Nurse Corps	Number of Awards
Distinguished Service Medal	1
Distinguished Flying Cross	2*
Silver Star	4
Legion of Merit	12
Soldiers Medal	5
Bronze Star (1 with Oak Leaf Cluster)	332
Air Medal (or Oak Leaf Cluster)	354
Citations	103
Purple Heart (1 with Oak Leaf Cluster)	60**
Total	873

1 awarded posthumously
**15 awarded posthumously*

A total of 201 Army nurses died during America's involvement in World War II, 92 of whom died in foreign theaters of war. In 1945, five nurses were still reported as missing in the Pacific area and another 26 nurses had been wounded in action.

Source: Facts About Nursing: The Nursing Information Bureau of the American Nurses' Association

Bibliography

Articles

Andrews, Gwen H. "Hospitalization Facilities for Women Veterans." American Journal of Nursing 45:10 (1945): 382-383.

Banfield, Gertrude S. "American Nurses - We Are At War!" American Journal of Nursing 42:4 (1942): 354-357.

_____. "This War - The Business of Every One of Us." American Journal of Nursing 42:10 (1942): 1126.

Beard, Mary. "The Mobilization of Nursing in National Defense." American Journal of Nursing 41:12 (1941): 1361-1364.

Beattie, Edith M. "Nurse Draft Legislation and the ANA - A Summary." American Journal of Nursing 45:7 (1945): 546-548.

Bernays, Edward L. "America Looks at Nursing." American Journal of Nursing 46:9 (1946): 590-592.

_____. "The Armed Forces and the Nursing Profession." American Journal of Nursing 46:3 (1946): 166-69.

_____. "Opinion Molders Appraise Nursing." American Journal of Nursing 45 (1945): 1005-1011.

_____. "A Public Relations Viewpoint." American Journal of Nursing 45:5 (1945): 351-353.

Clarke, Alice R. "Thirty-Seven Months as a POW." American Journal of Nursing 45:5 (1945): 342-345.

Clayton, Frederick. "Front Line Surgical Nurses." American Journal of Nursing 44:3 (1944): 234-235.

_____. "An Evacuation Unit Serves Under Fire." American Journal of Nursing 44:5 (1944):453-455.

Darnton, E. "Army Nurse Trains for Battle." N.Y. Times Magazine October 24, 1943: 18-19.

Day, Frank. "Justice For Army and Navy Nurses." American Journal of Nursing 43:8 (1943): 703.

Engel, D.D. "I Was Married in Battle." American Magazine October, 1942: 112-116.

Goostray, Stella. "The League Considers Defense." American Journal of Nursing 41:7 (1941): 816-832.

_____. "Supply, Demand, and Standards." American Journal of Nursing 41:6 (1941): 745-747.

Grayson, Frances. "War and Nursing." American Journal of Nursing 44:8 (1944): 788.

Jose, Mary. "Some Army Nurses' Postwar Plans." American Journal of Nursing 45:8 (1945): 596-597.

Kirk, Norman T. "Girls in the Foxholes." American Magazine May, 1944: 17, 94-97.

Marley, Faye. "Training Nurses For War." Hygeia November, 1943: 788-789.

Martin, Pete. "Angels in Long Underwear" Saturday Evening Post July 31, 1943: 9-11.

McGuire, S.H. and Dorothy W. Conrad. "Postwar Plans of Army & Navy Nurses." American Journal of Nursing 46 (1946): 305-6 and 45 (1945): 1021-23.

"Mortality Statistics for Nurses in the Armed Forces" American Journal of Nursing 45 (1945): p. 576.

Mountin, Joseph. "Nursing - A Critical Analysis." American Journal of Nursing 43:1 (1943): 29-34.

_____. "Suggestions to Nurses on Postwar Adjustments." American Journal of Nursing 44:4 91944): 321-325.

"The Nurses' Contribution to American Victory: Facts & Figures From Pearl Harbor to V-J Day" American Journal of Nursing 45 (1945): 683-86.

"The Nurses Have Not Lagged Behind." Saturday Evening Post April 28, 1945: 108.

Paxton, Vincoe. "With the Field Hospital Nurses in Germany: Army Nurses Serve Forward Combat Units." American Journal of Nursing 45:2 (1945): 131-133.

Randolph, Mary Walker. "What the Army Expects from the Profession." American Journal of Nursing 46:2 (1946): 95-97.

Sharritt, Edna E. "Where Are the Ex-Service Nurses?" American Journal of Nursing 46 (1946): 849-51.

Stewart, Isabel. "Nursing Preparedness: Some Lessons from World War I." American Journal of Nursing 41:7 (1941): 804-815.

Stimson, Julia C. "Our Hour." American Journal of Nursing 42:2 (1942): 140.

Tead, O.W. "The Development of Leadership Power."
American Journal of Nursing 42:8 (1942): 867.

Valentine, E.R. "Nurses on the Fronts." N.Y. Times
Magazine September, 1942: 12-18, 53.

White, Ruth Y. "At Anzio Beach." American Journal of
Nursing 44:4 91944): pp. 370-371.

Wickenden, Elmira B. "The National Nursing Council
Reports." American Journal of Nursing 43:9 (1943): 808.

Williams, Anne K. "Patriotism Is Not Enough." American
Journal of Nursing 41:3 (1941): 297-298.

Worcester, D.A. "Leadership." American Journal of
Nursing 41:3 (1941): 280-284.

Books

American Institute of Public Opinion. The Gallup Poll:
Public Opinion, 1935-1971. N.Y.: Random House, 1972.

Anderson, Karen. Wartime Women: Sex Roles, Family
Relations, and the Status of Women During World War II.
Westport CT: Greenwood Press, 1981.

Archard, Theresa. G.I. Nightingale: The Story of an
American Army Nurse. N.Y.: W.W. Norton & Co., Inc.,
1945.

Aynes, Edith A. From Nightingale to Eagle: An Army
Nurse's History. Englewood Cliffs: Prentice-Hall, Inc.,
1973.

Bingham, Stella. Ministering Angels. Oradell, N.J.:
Medical Economics Co., 1979.

214

Bledstein, Burton J. The Culture of Professionalism: The Middle Class and the Development of Higher Education. New York: W.W. Norton, & Co., 1976.

Bullough, Vern, et. al. American Nursing: A Bibliographical Dictionary. New York: Garland Publishing, Inc., 1988.

Campbell, D'Ann. Women at War with America: Private Lives in a Patriotic Era. Cambridge: Harvard University Press, 1984.

Cantril, Hadley and Mildred Strunk (eds.) Public Opinion, 1935-1946. Princeton Press, 1951.

Cohen, Helen A. The Nurses Quest for a Professional Identity. Menlo Park, CA: Addison-Wesley Publishing Co., 1981.

Dietz, Lena Dixon. History and Modern Nursing. Philadelphia: F.A. Davis Co., 1963.

Dolan, Josephine A. Goodnow's History of Nursing. Philadelphia: W.B. Saunders Co., 1963.

Ehrenreich, Barbara and Deirdre English. Witches, midwives, and nurses: A History of Women Healers. Old Westbury, N.Y.: The Feminist Press, 1973.

Enloe, Cynthia. Does Khaki Become You? The Militarization of Women's Lives. Boston: South End Press, 1983.

Etzioni, Amitai, ed. The Semi-Professions and Their Organization: Teachers, Nurses, Social Workers. New York: The Free Press, 1969.

Faderman, Lillian. Odd Girls and Twilight Lovers: A History of Lesbian Life in Twentieth Century America. New York: Columbia University Press, 1991.

Flikke, Julia O. Nurses in Action: A Story of the Army Nurse Corps. Philadelphia: J.B. Lippincott Co., 1943.

Hartmann, Susan M. The Homefront and Beyond: American Women in the 1940s. Boston: Twayne Publishing, 1982.

Hine, Darlene Clark. "Mable Staupers and the Integration of Black Nurses into the Armed Forces." Women and Health in America. Ed. Judith Walzer Leavitt. Madison: University of Wisconsin Press, 1984.

Kalisch, Philip A. and Beatrice J. Kalisch. The Advance of American Nursing. Boston: Little, Brown and Co., 1986.

_____. The Changing Image of the Nurse. Menlo Park: CA: Addison-Wesley, 1987.

Kaufman, Martin, ed., Dictionary of American Nursing Biography. New York: Greenwood Press, 1988.

Leavitt, Judith W., ed. Women and Health in America. Madison: University of Wisconsin, 1984.

Melosh, Barbara. "The Physicians' Hand:" Work Culture and Conflict in American Nursing. Philadelphia: Temple University Press, 1982.

Nursing Information Bureau of the American Nursing Association. Facts About Nursing. New York, Volumes 1939-1950.

Piemonte, Robert V. and Cindy Gurney, eds. Highlights in the History of the Army Nurse Corps. Washington, D.C.: U.S. Dept. of the Army, Military History, 1987.

Redmond, Juanita. I Served on Bataan. N.Y.: Garland Publishing, Inc., 1943.

Reverby, Susan M. The History of American Nursing. N.Y.: Garland Publishing, Inc., 1984.

_____. Ordered to Care: The Dilemma of American Nursing, 1850-1955. Cambridge: Cambridge University Press, 1987.

Risch, Erma and Chester L. Kieffer. United States Army in World War II - The Technical Services: The Quartermaster Corps: Organization, Supply, and Services. Vol. II. Washington, D.C.: Office of Military History, Dept. of the Army, 1955.

Roberts, Mary M., American Nursing: History and Interpretation. N.Y.: Macmillan, 1954.

Rosenberg, Charles E., The Care of Strangers: The Rise of America's Hospital System. New York: Basic Books, Inc., 1987.

Smith, Clarence McKittrick. United States Army in World War II - The Technical Services: The Medical Department: Hospital and Evacuation in the Zone of Interior. Vol.6. Washington, D.C.: Office of Military History, Dept. of the Army, 1956.

Summers, Anne. Angels and Citizens: British Women as Military Nurses, 1854-1914. London: Routledge and Kegan Paul, 1988.

Treadwell, Mattie E. United States Army in World War II
-The Women's Army Corps. Vol.14. Washington, D.C.:
Office of Military History, Dept. of the Army, 1954.

Tomes, Nancy. "'Little World of Our Own': The
Pennsylvania Hospital Training School for Nurses,
1895-1907." Women and Health in America. Ed. Judith
Walzer Leavitt. Madison: University of Wisconsin Press,
1984.

Vicinus, Martha. Independent Women: Work and
Community for Single Women, 1850-1920. Chicago:
University of Chicago Press, 1985.

Vollmer, H.M. and D.L. Mills. Professionalization.
Englewood Cliffs: Prentice-Hall, Inc., 1966.

Wiltse, Charles M. United States Army in World War II -
The Technical Services: The Medical Department:
Medical Service in the Mediterranean and Minor Theaters.
9Vol.6. Washington, D.C.: Office of Military History,
Dept. of the Army, 1965.

Unpublished Manuscripts

Blackwelder, Julia K. "Motherhood and Women's Work
in Cold War America." Unpublished article, 1992.

Kanneberg, Lisa A. "From World War to Cold War:
Women Electrical Workers and Their Union, 1940-1955."
M.A. Thesis. University of North Carolina at Charlotte,
1990.

Light, Dorothy Chinnis. Personal Diary. April 13, 1943 -
    March 26, 1946.

Interviews/Correspondence

Light, Dorothy Chinnis. Recorded Interview. July 1990.

Parsons, Dorothy. Letter to the author. January 31, 1991.

_____. Letter to the author. May 2, 1991.

A

Aachen, Germany, 102
A-Bag, 90
ACTH, 31
Ad Council, 75
Advertising, 50, 66, 75, 186
Age, 20, 27, 58, 63, 118, 187, 201
Albania, 102
Alcohol, 115
Allowances, 85
AMA, American Medical Association, 51, 180
American College of Surgeons, 173
American Journal of Nursing, 27, 28, 35, 46, 59, 97, 169, 198, 211, 212, 213, 214
American Medical Association [AMA], 173, 174
American Nurses Association [ANA], 12, 19, 28, 44, 45, 144, 190
American Nursing History and Interpretation, 28, 217
American Red Cross, 13, 24, 27, 45, 48, 50, 54, 60, 66, 72, 75, 76, 153, 178, 198, 200
American Red Cross Nursing Service [ARCNS], 24, 45, 48, 178, 198, 200
ANA, American Nurses Association, 12, 22, 29, 45, 70, 71, 142, 143, 145, 150, 153, 154, 165, 168, 176, 191, 201, 204, 211
ANC, Army Nurse Corps, 12, 21, 68, 86, 132, 133, 152, 178
Andrew Jergens, 75
Anzio Beach, 214
Archard, Theresa, 57, 91

ARCNS, American Red Cross Nursing Service, 24, 45
Army Medical Service, 12
Army Nurse Corps [ANC], 12, 18, 19, 20, 34, 37, 43, 44, 48, 56, 57, 58, 64, 66, 72, 75, 77, 83, 84, 87, 96, 112, 113, 134, 145, 152, 158, 177, 188, 198, 200, 201, 210, 216, 217
Army Postal Service, 107
Army School of Nursing, 25, 27
Army School of Nursing at Camp Sherman - Ohio, 27
Army, United States, 21, 110, 148
Art of Caring, 181
Association of Collegiate Schools of Nursing, 29, 198
Augustana Hospital Training School - Chicago, 20
Aynes, Edith, 56

B

Base Hospital, 15
Bataan, 79, 217
Battle Fatigue, 161
Battle of the Bulge, 68
B-Bag, 90
Beard, Mary, 18, 24, 45, 197
Benefits, 32, 85, 146, 150, 151, 168, 178, 189
Bernays, Edward, 154, 171
Billets, 89
Bivouac, 87
Blanchfield, Florence A., 18, 21
Blood Banks, 31
Boston University, 23

C

Cadet Nurse Corps, 25, 27
Calisthenics, 87, 92

223

Public Health, 29, 197, 198,
  203
Public Opinion, 199, 214, 215
Public Relations, 211
PX, Post Exchange, 95, 96

Q

Quartermaster General, 96
Quinine, 31, 65
Quota, 42, 50, 76, 187

R

Ravenel, France, 121
Ravenel, South Carolina, 58
Recreation, 105, 170
Recruitment efforts, 42, 46,
  187
Recruits, 42, 45, 53, 76, 86,
  186
Red Cross Nurses' Club, 105
Red Cross Nursing Service,
  14, 24, 29, 56, 67
relative rank, 21, 85
Rensselaer Polytechnic
  Institute, 46
Report of Separation, 151
Reputation, 115
Reserves, 54, 58, 145, 201
Resolutions, 165
Respect, 112, 153, 164, 173,
  178, 189, 194
Rest, 59, 84, 105, 110, 149,
  160
Restrictions, age, 187
Restrictions, marriage, 63
RN, Registered Nurse, 148,
  197, 198
Roberts, Mary, 18, 27, 46, 169
Rock of Gibraltar, 92
Rockefeller Foundation, 26
Romance, 121
Roosevelt, Eleanor, 60
Roosevelt, President, 68, 108
Rotary Club, 51
Rumors, 43

S

Safety, 30, 43, 91, 106, 135,
  187
Salary, 32, 56, 163, 164, 166,
  167, 168, 176
Scholarships, 51
Scotland, 92
Scutari, 9
Selective Service Act, 61, 69
Selective Training and Service
  Act, 150
Self-sacrifice, 18, 45, 84
Semi-Professions, 6, 7, 180
Senate Committee on Military
  Affairs, 72
Separation Orders, 151
Service Extension Act, 150
Sex Objects, 116
Shaver, Dorothy, 96
shell shock, 15
Shifts, 62, 98
Sidney, Texas, 117
Sight-seeing, 105
Slander, 112
Social Security, 143
Southside Hospital Training
  School for Nurses -
  Pittsburg, 21
Spelhaug, First Lieutenant
  Glenda, 117
Standard Oil, 46
Stark General Hospital -
  Charleston, SC, 105
Station Hospital, 58th, 92
Status, 4, 5, 7, 8, 12, 19, 21,
  24, 31, 33, 34, 40, 41, 65,
  79, 85, 89, 109, 136, 142,
  146, 147, 149, 153, 154,
  165, 168, 171, 172, 173,
  175, 180, 186, 189, 191,
  192, 193
Stimson, Julia C., 18, 197, 198
Strategy, 52, 78, 85, 103, 111,
  154
Sulfanilamide, 31
Sullivan, Margaret, 54

Y

Yale University, 17

About the Author

Marsha Burris holds a Master of Arts degree in History. She lives in Charlotte, North Carolina where she is Adjunct Professor in History at the University of North Carolina at Charlotte. Her academic fields of interest include Twentieth Century British History, Women's Contributions to World War II, and Ancient and Medieval Medicine.

The author invites your comments and questions at:

ML_BURRIS@yahoo.com

www.ingramcontent.com/pod-product-compliance
Lightning Source LLC
Chambersburg PA
CBHW031950080426
42735CB00007B/341